PAIN AND EMOTION

PAIN
AND
EMOTION

BY

ROGER TRIGG

CLARENDON PRESS · OXFORD
1970

Oxford University Press, Ely House, London W. 1

GLASGOW NEW YORK TORONTO MELBOURNE WELLINGTON
CAPE TOWN SALISBURY IBADAN NAIROBI LUSAKA ADDIS ABABA
BOMBAY CALCUTTA MADRAS KARACHI LAHORE DACCA
KUALA LUMPUR SINGAPORE HONG KONG TOKYO

PRINTED IN GREAT BRITAIN
AT THE UNIVERSITY PRESS
ABERDEEN

ACKNOWLEDGEMENTS

I AM greatly indebted to Mrs. P. R. Foot and to Professor G. Ryle for their help and kind encouragement. I have profited enormously from the criticism and many valuable suggestions which they have offered. I must also thank others with whom I have discussed some of the topics of this book. I am particularly grateful to Professor R. M. Hare, Dr. A. Kenny, Mr. C. C. W. Taylor, and Mr. J. O. Urmson.

R.H.T.

CONTENTS

I

IS PAIN A SENSATION?

1. *Pleasure and Pain*

IT seems obvious that pain is a sensation, but this has been regularly challenged. Some philosophers have emphasized the similarity of pain to the emotions. They have been tempted to classify it as one or to put it in a special category on its own somewhere between sensation and emotion. Wittgenstein[1] notes that pain is differentiated from other sensations by what he calls a 'characteristic expression'. He says of pain[2]:

This concept resembles that of e.g. tactile sensation (through the characteristics of localization, genuine duration, intensity, quality) and at the same time that of the emotions through its expression (facial expressions, gestures, noises).

Philosophers and psychologists turned to this problem towards the end of the nineteenth century, when advances in physiology seemed to show that pain was a specific sense linked to a specific nerve path. F. H. Bradley wrote[3] that 'not a pleasure but something pleasant is what we experience'—and he would have said that we do not experience pain but only something painful. The assumption that pain and pleasure must be treated in the same way lay behind everything that was said at this period, and was usually stated explicitly.

H. R. Marshall followed Bradley in denying that pain was a sensation. He maintained that the pain of a cut or burn could always be analysed into a tactile or a temperature sensation and a feeling of displeasure. He says bluntly[4]: 'I draw no distinctions other than those of degree or breadth between pain and disagreeableness or between pleasure and agreeableness.' His is primarily a theory of displeasure, and it is

[1] Zettel, § 483.
[2] op. cit. § 485.
[3] 'On Pleasure, Pain, Desire and Volition', *Mind*, xiii (1888), 2.
[4] *Pain, Pleasure and Aesthetics*, p. 6.

conditioned very largely by a desire to keep the concepts of pain and pleasure parallel. He wants to vindicate the 'judgement of common sense' and he puts this as follows[1]:

Pleasure and pain are two states which are too disparate to be commonly known by any one word, but so inseparably connected that they must be mentioned in one breath. This community of character should seemingly lead us to hold that where we class the one we must class the other also . . . It seems to me clear from common speech that the ordinary man naturally thinks of pain as a sensation and of pleasure as an emotion. This fact . . . serves to cast doubt upon any view which would class pleasure and pain exclusively with sensation, as it also does upon one which would class them exclusively with emotion.

The view which Bradley and Marshall put forward became known as the 'aspect theory' from their opinion that pleasure and pain were mere aspects of experiences. The pain of a sprained ankle and the pain of bereavement were both analysed in the same way. Both experiences would be 'coloured' by displeasure. In the ankle case the sensation would not be pain, any more than the bare knowledge of bereavement is pain. According to the theory, both carry with them a quality or 'tone' of pain.

All attempts to keep the balance between pleasure and pain came to nothing in the face of the clear distinction made by Henry Head between 'discomfort' and 'pain'.[2] He claimed:

Pain is a distinct sensory quality equivalent to hot and cold and its intensity can be roughly graded according to the force expended in stimulation. Discomfort, on the other hand, is that feeling-tone which is directly opposed to pleasure. It may accompany sensations not in themselves essentially painful, as, for instance, that produced by tickling the sole of the foot.

This division between the emotional and sensational elements in the concept of pain, with the word 'pain' being reserved for the latter, met with immediate acceptance. Russell[3] said: 'We may use "pain" as the opposite of "pleasure" and "painful" as the opposite of "pleasant" or we may use "pain" to mean a certain sort of sensation, on a level with

---

[1] *Pain, Pleasure and Aesthetics*, p. 15.   [2] *Studies in Neurology*, p. 665.
[3] *The Analysis of Mind*, p. 70.

the sensations of heat and cold and touch. The latter use of the word has prevailed in psychological literature and it is now no longer used as the opposite of "pleasure".'

It seemed that any link between the concepts of pain and pleasure had been finally broken, and that pain had been finally classified as a sensation pure and simple. In fact in a textbook[1] revised in 1958 the authors still felt themselves able to talk of 'pathways for pain' and to state that 'pain is a specific sensory experience mediated through its own nerve structures'. Contemporary physiologists, however, realize that this is to underestimate the complexity of the phenomena accompanying the pain experience. It is also to make the mistake of thinking that a single nerve-impulse or a collection of impulses *is* a pain, whereas it is now realized that the job of such impulses is to carry information to the brain to be 'decoded'. As physiologists discover more about the brain and its function, they are placing less emphasis on the role of nerves and the signals they convey and more on the importance of the interpretation of the signals by the brain.

This change in the scientific view of pain and the increasing emphasis on the emotional elements in pain is not unnaturally having its effect on philosophers and psychologists. A. R. Manser[2] notes that 'experimental psychologists are now finding that the old idea that pain consisted in the stimulation of "pain-nerves" is not altogether satisfactory'. He criticizes Ryle,[3] who claims that ' "Pain", in the sense in which I have pains in my stomach, is not the opposite of "pleasure". In this sense, a pain is a sensation of a special sort, which we ordinarily dislike having'. Manser says of this kind of account,[4]

It fails to indicate what seems to be the most important quality of pain, its unpleasantness or its 'to-be-avoidedness'. For that something will be painful is, other things being equal, a perfectly good reason to avoid it. But is it the sensation itself which is to be avoided, or the unpleasantness of the sensation? Most modern philosophers seem to ignore this question, to use 'pain' for a sensation which is

---

[1] Wolff and Wolf, *Pain*, p. 8.
[2] 'Pleasure', *Proceedings of the Aristotelian Society*, lxi (1960–1), 224–5.
[3] *Concept of Mind*, p. 109.
[4] op. cit. p. 224.

to be avoided. This has an obvious disadvantage in that it leaves no word to describe the opposite of pleasure, those things which, although not giving rise to painful sensations, are nevertheless to be avoided.

Like the aspect theorists, Manser is drawn towards equating pain with displeasure, as also is a psychologist, M. D. Arnold, who in a recent book[1] has said that the extremes of pleasant feelings may be called 'pleasure', those of unpleasant feelings, 'pain'.

Any theory which, like the aspect theory, keeps the concepts of pain and pleasure on the same footing by denying that pain is a sensation will claim that 'mental' and 'physical' pain are identical. Pains, it will say, are not sensations, although we may find some sensations painful, just as we find some thoughts painful. In his article on 'Pleasure'[2] C. C. W. Taylor does in fact say precisely this. 'The things which we find painful', he asserts, 'include both sensations and situations, encounters, discoveries and the like, but finding any of these painful is not itself having any bodily sensations. So pain is not a sensation, but *a* pain may be sensation.'

The aspect theorists denied that pain was actually an emotion even though they equated it with extreme displeasure. They thought of pain and pleasure as qualities of experiences, including emotions. However, their denial that pain is a sensation leads very naturally to the view that it is an emotion. This is a very easy step to take if 'displeasure' is regarded as a rough synonym for distress.

To define pain as an emotion is to dismiss the view of the ordinary man that pain is something he feels at different places in his body. Just as one would feel the emotion of distress at someone's unkind words, so, it is claimed, to have a pain in one's foot is to feel extreme displeasure or distress at a sensation in one's foot. This does have the very definite advantage of suggesting that the words 'pain' and 'painful' are not being used in two different senses according to whether they are referring to sensations or more general mental experiences. For if we insist on the common-sense view that 'pain' is the name of a particular kind of sensation (or class of sensations),

[1] *Emotion and Personality*, i. 19.
[2] *Analysis* 23 (Supplement), 1963, p. 10.

we have to admit that reference to, for example, a 'painful interview' involves an analogical use of the word. To be involved in such an interview is not usually to suffer sensations of an unpleasant kind. It is rather to be distressed by the occasion, and by our use of the word 'painful' we are on this view making a comparison between our distress at the interview and our feelings when we are in pain.

With the analysis of physical pain as 'distress at a sensation', one does not have to be too worried about any apparent sensational elements of pain. The localization of pain presents no problem. It is, one can say, not the pain but the sensation which distresses us that we localize. Similarly the fact that we cannot even be said to be in pain unless we feel a sensation of some sort need only illustrate the truth that to be distressed we must be distressed *by* something. Otherwise this might seem to drive a wedge between pain and an emotion like anger. Like the emotions, pain has its characteristic outward expression, but internally, if we equated sensations of pain with the feelings we usually have when angry, differences immediately appear. 'I am in (physical) pain' entails 'I feel pain'—or, to keep consistent with the 'aspect theory', 'I feel a painful sensation'. Unfelt pain is a contradiction. It is however by no means obvious that 'I am angry' or 'I am afraid' entails 'I feel angry' or 'I feel afraid'. These emotions do have characteristic feelings and we talk of 'waves of anger' coming over us, but the concepts do not require the feelings to be present all the time. I can be angry for a whole week without feeling angry for every moment, but I can't be in pain for that time without feeling pain continuously.

2. *The 'Intentionality' of Pain*

One of the prime characteristics of all emotions is that they essentially have 'objects'. In other words, one is naturally angry at or afraid of *something* and never just angry or afraid. I must be disgusted by something, proud of something, hate some person or thing and so on. However, must I necessarily be anxious about something? Cannot I be in a general state of anxiety without being anxious about anything in particular? I can be depressed at something, but may not I sometimes merely be depressed? Cannot I be generally cheerful or happy without being cheerful or happy at anything? Philosophers often treat this kind of question as a challenge to the view that emotions have 'objects' and sometimes respond by dogmatically insisting that, if there is no particular 'object', there must be a general one such as 'life' or 'everything'. There is an element of truth in this, but unfortunately these look rather spurious 'objects' which seem to have been produced merely to save the theory.

Although 'anxiety' and 'depression' often function as names for particular emotions it does not necessarily follow that they always do. In fact, in so far as we talk readily of being in an anxious mood or a depressed state, it looks as if we should recognize that they are often names of moods and not emotions. The same is true of other states which appear to be like emotions but have no particular 'object'. I can be in a cheerful mood or a happy one. I can have a mood of elation and so on. If these are moods, it is hardly surprising that they do not exemplify the normal pattern for an emotion.

If I am in an irritable mood, I am liable to become angry at things which I would normally accept with equanimity. In other words, irritability is a disposition to experience a particular emotion. It is not, however, possible to make all moods parasitic on the concept of emotion in this way. If I am in a frivolous mood, I am not prone to undergo a particular emotion. I see everything in a much less serious light than usual and will act accordingly. If I am in a happy mood, I feel as if everything is going well; I take a more optimistic view of things than usual. If my mood is one of depression, the reverse is true; I am inclined to take a gloomy view of everything. This may not necessarily mean that I get into a series of emotional states. Indeed, I may merely fail to get excited or pleased about a piece of news which would usually thrill me. I might not get amused at something I usually found funny. In fact, words for moods indicate the general 'climate' of my thought at a particular time, while words which refer to emotions merely describe particular squalls.

The 'objects' of emotions such as fear and anger are not usually sensations. Even if we are afraid that a certain pang we feel is an indication of heart trouble, it is not the pang that we are afraid of, but its imagined significance. It is true

that we might sometimes fear a pain *per se*, because, for instance, we known we might not be able to bear it. In general,
however, the presence of a sensation is not necessary for
emotion. 'Distress' (or 'pain', if it is an emotion) is a major
exception. We often are distressed at sensations. The main
difference between 'mental pain' and 'physical pain' could well
be the type of 'object' which each has. 'Mental pain' could be
distress at situations, while 'physical pain' would be distress at
sensations. It need not be at all surprising in that case that it
is logically necessary for someone suffering 'physical pain' to
feel something. If the sensation was absent, there would be no
'object' for the emotion, and hence no pain. Anger, on the
other hand, may still have an 'object', whether the feelings
often associated with it are present or not.

A similar combination of circumstances does not quite give
us equivalent certainty about 'physical' pain. Here the presence of a sensation is all-important, and only the patient
himself can tell us of it. In a paradigm case of pain, when
someone is writhing in apparent agony with a gaping wound,
there can not only still be a logical doubt but even a very
real doubt as to whether the man is in pain. H. K. Beecher[1]
said of men wounded in battle that 'patients are described as
"writhing in pain" and large doses of morphine administered
when the real problem is restlessness from cerebral anoxia or
excitement from fear and apprehension'—and that this was
the case was shown by the fact that sedatives had far more
effect than morphine.

Any attempt to assimilate 'physical' to 'mental' pain cannot,
as we have seen, allow painful sensations to be regarded in the
same light as feelings of anger. G. E. Moore saw that they are
even different from painful thoughts. He says[2]:

Generally when you have a sensation that is painful, in any marked
degree, you also desire to be rid of the sensation in question. . . .
Whether the same is true of painful thoughts, I doubt, e.g. when the
thought of some foolish or awkward thing you have done or said is
painful to you, you don't seem to desire to be rid of the thought;
what you desire (if anything) is that you had not said or done the
thing.

[1] 'Pain in Men Wounded in Battle', *Annals of Surgery*, 123, 1946.
[2] *Commonplace Book*, p. 31.

Moore is in effect drawing attention to the kind of 'object' the emotion of distress (or pain) takes. He talks of 'a desire to be rid of something', but such a desire must be a part of the concept of distress. It would be extremely odd if someone claimed to be distressed by an event or a sensation, but, other things being equal, was quite happy to continue in his predicament. This lack of any desire to be extricated from the situation would make us doubt his claim.

Whereas the 'object' of our distress when we are suffering physical pain is a sensation, and we talk of 'painful sensations' or 'sensations of pain', our everyday talk of 'painful thoughts' should not be taken to imply that our thoughts are the 'object' of our distress. The situations about which we think are the true 'objects', and our thoughts are the indispensable means by which we become aware of their significance. It is necessarily true that we cannot be distressed by something if we are not aware of it. To be distressed, however, by something which we think about is very different from being distressed by our thoughts. We can be distressed at a bereavement without being distressed at the fact that we are thinking about it. It is true that the situation which so disturbs us may be an imagined one. The person may not in fact be dead, for example. Even then it is not our thought that distresses us; it is what we imagine to be the case. If we find out our mistake, our mental anguish will leave us, no matter how much thinking we do.

Does the emotion involved in physical pain fit in with this pattern? Taking 'pain' to refer to an emotion, can there be pain at a non-existent sensation? Or, taking it as a sensation, can we feel distress at a non-existent pain? The short answer is that sensations, including painful ones, logically must be felt. An unfelt sensation is not a sensation at all. What of the well-known case of someone flinching under a dentist's drill, apparently in pain, when the drill has not yet touched him? If asked, the patient would claim that he had felt pain, and his emotional anguish would be genuine enough. When told that the drill had not touched him, he might withdraw his claim and admit that the 'object' of his distress was the general threatening situation and his expectation of pain. If, however, he insisted he had felt pain, we are in no position to contradict him on the grounds that there was no apparent physical cause. Ultimately only he can tell us whether he was in pain or not. We must conclude that either the 'object' of his anguish is not a painful sensation but something more general or that he is actually having a sensation. The possibility of distress directed at a sensation which is only imaginary cannot arise.

3. *Intentional Verbs and Objects*

We cannot feel distress at a non-existent sensation. If we are distressed by our pain, it looks as if we must actually have a pain. This suggests that the emotion normally involved in physical pain fails to conform with the usual pattern of what has been termed 'intentionality'. The possible non-existence of the object seems to be a mark of many 'intentional' verbs, and Miss Anscombe makes it one of their defining features,[1] together with the 'non-substitutability of the different descriptions of the object, where it does exist' and the 'possible indeterminacy of the object'. To take the example of fear, I can be afraid of 'the man next door' when no one lives there. If someone does occupy the house, I need not fear him under the description 'headmaster of such and such a school', even if that description is true of him. I can, finally, have only a very vague idea of him and can think of him without, for example, thinking of him as having any particular height. This last criterion is closely linked with the second. These are grammatical criteria, and Miss Anscombe explicitly defines intentional objects as 'the sub-class of direct objects characterized by these three connected features'.

Chisholm[2] makes a similar attempt to find criteria 'by means of which', he says, 'we can distinguish sentences that are intentional, or are used intentionally, in a certain language from sentences that are not'. He suggests three 'marks of intentionality'. He maintains first of all that a sentence is intentional, 'if it uses a substantial expression—a name or a description—in such a way that neither the sentence nor its contradictory implies either that there is or that there isn't anything to which the substantival expression truly applies'.

---

[1] G. E. M. Anscombe, 'The Intentionality of Sensation', *Analytical Philosophy*, ed. R. J. Butler (second series), pp. 161–2.
[2] *Perceiving*, p. 170.

This is equivalent to Miss Anscombe's first criterion. With his second 'mark', Chisholm extends this to cover propositions. He writes: 'Secondly, let us say, of any noncompound sentence which contains a propositional clause, that it is intentional provided that neither the sentence nor its contradictory implies either that the propositional clause is true or that it is false.' On this criterion, the sentence 'I am afraid that the man next door will sue me' is intentional. The mere existence of my fear does not entail that what I am afraid of will happen. Similarly, it is an unfortunate fact of life that if I believe that something is so, it does not necessarily follow that it is. Chisholm's third 'mark' is the same as Miss Anscombe's second. I can know who the Prime Minister is and hold very definite opinions about his capabilities, while claiming to be completely ignorant of the qualities of 'the M.P. for such and such a constituency', even when (as I fail to realize) the Prime Minister is that member. This feature is what Quine terms 'referential opacity'.

What is the point of talking about intentionality? The whole notion was re-introduced into philosophy as a means of distinguishing the mental and the physical. Brentano[1] followed the medieval scholastics and emphasized that every mental phenomenon is characterized by the intentional inexistence of an object, 'and', he says, 'what we would call, although in not entirely unambiguous terms, the reference to a content, a direction upon an object'. By way of illustration he says: 'In judgement something is affirmed or denied, in love something is loved, in hate something is hated, in desire something is desired, etc.' He concludes: 'This intentional inexistence is exclusively characteristic of mental phenomena. No physical phenomenon manifests anything similar. Consequently, we can define mental phenomena by saying that they are such phenomena as include an object intentionally within themselves.' Brentano recognizes that pleasure and pain present him with a difficulty. They appear to be mental phenomena, and yet it had been alleged that they do not take intentional objects. Brentano has no difficulty in showing that this is just not true in many cases. He points out: 'We say that a person

---

[1] 'The Distinction between Mental and Physical Phenomena', trans. by D. B. Terrell in *Realism and the Background of Phenomenology*, Ed. R. M. Chisholm, p. 50.

rejoices in or about something, that a person sorrows or grieves about something. And once again: that delights me, that pains me, that hurts me and so on.' He admits that his analysis is more difficult with ordinary physical pain, such as that aroused by a cut or a burn, but, as we shall see, he insists that even in that case there is both a 'physical' and a 'mental' element.

It is crucial to distinguish the cause of an emotion from its 'object', and it would be very valuable if we could find criteria which would distinguish the one from the other. Indigestion can be the cause of a businessman's anger, but he may be angry with his secretary rather than his indigestion. This distinction can get blurred. Brentano passes from talking about what delights me to what hurts me. The former is more likely to be an 'object' than the latter. I can be hurt by a slight and this means I am distressed at it. On the other hand, I can be hurt by a stone and this means that the stone has caused me pain. In the first case I must be aware of the slight. In the second I need only be aware of the pain. We do not always know the cause of a pain. Kenny tries to distinguish between pain and the emotions by saying[1]: 'It is possible to be in pain without knowing what is hurting one, as it is not possible to be delighted without knowing what is delighting one.' This comparison does not distinguish between pain and delight as it was intended to, as there is a shift in it from cause to 'object'. It is certainly not possible to be delighted without being delighted at something—without an 'object' of one's delight. It is possible to be delighted without knowing the *cause* of one's delight. I could be delighted at a business proposal without realizing that the cause of my delight is the good meal I have just eaten. Our ignorance about causes puts delight and pain on exactly the same footing. Only if pain does not have an 'object' can it be distinguished from the emotions as Kenny was trying to do.

Are the criteria proposed by Chisholm and Miss Anscombe adequate to distinguish 'objects' from causes? Do they enable us to separate mental from physical phenomena? 'Intentional inexistence' has been regarded as the crucial mark of intentionality, and yet there do appear to be psychological verbs

[1] *Action Emotion and Will*, p. 60.

which presuppose the existence of their objects, as well as
non-psychological verbs which in some sentences imply neither
the existence nor the non-existence of their objects. If it is
true that I know John Smith, then John Smith must exist. If
he doesn't, I clearly cannot know him. Similarly if it is true
that I know that the Queen of the United Kingdom is also
Queen of Australia, it follows that the Queen *is* also Queen of
Australia. I could not know that she was the Queen of India
as she is not. In other words, 'know' entails the existence of the
object known or the truth of the proposition known and by two
of the criteria proposed cannot be an intentional verb. On the
other hand it clearly is according to the criterion of the 'non-
substitutability of different descriptions of the object'. Someone
who was ignorant of Commonwealth constitutions could
intelligibly claim to know that the Queen of England lives in
London but deny that this was true of the Queen of Australia.
It looks as if 'intentional inexistence' cannot be a necessary
condition of intentionality.

'Know' is not the only counter-example. I cannot recognize
someone who does not exist. If I recognize the man who is
Prime Minister, that man must exist. There is always a
possibility of misdescription. A visitor to England might
claim to have recognized the 'British President' and be told
that it was the Prime Minister. It is nevertheless still true that
he recognized him under some description. In the same way I
might recognize someone under one description and not under
another. I can recognize the man I met last week without
realizing he was the mayor. Chisholm's second criterion must
also be challenged. I can recognize truths but if it is true that
I recognize them it follows that they are truths. If I recognize
that I broke the law, I must have broken the law. The same
applies with 'realize'. If I realize that I exceeded the speed
limit, I did exceed the speed limit. 'Enjoy' is a further example.
I must be enjoying something which exists, even if I have a
wrong conception of it. Oedipus could enjoy marrying
Jocasta without necessarily enjoying marrying his mother.
Nevertheless, neither he nor anyone else could enjoy what
was only a figment of their imagination. They could enjoy
imagining something, but that is a different case. A further
batch of examples might be provided by verbs of perception.

It is certainly often held[1] that 'see', 'hear', 'smell' and so on,
only record successes. If I see something, the thing must exist.
Otherwise I can only say that I thought I saw it.

Is 'intentional inexistence' a sufficient condition for intentionality? I might boast 'my car can outstrip any sportscar in
town' without implying that there necessarily are any sports
models in the town. All I am saying is that if there are, my car
is faster than them. According to this criterion, the sentence
ought to be intentional. It looks as if the possible non-existence
of an object is neither a necessary nor a sufficient condition for
intentionality. It might be objected that the superficial
grammar of the sentence is misleading and that it is of the
logical form: For all x, if x is a sportscar in this town, my car
can outstrip it. This is completely irrelevant. Miss Anscombe
and Chisholm are quite explicitly looking at English sentences
and the direct objects in them in a quest for *grammatical*
criteria for intentionality. If their criteria let in sentences
which contain no psychological verbs and which we have no
wish to call intentional, the criteria must be inadequate.

Chisholm's second condition, which applied the criterion of
intentional inexistence to propositions, seems to meet the same
kind of difficulty. Counter-examples have indicated that it is
not necessary. Can it be regarded as sufficient? A political
commentator might say: 'The Prime Minister will do whatever will bring him victory in the next election.' This could
well be true whether there is anything which would bring him
victory or not. If there was, he would do it. The commentator
could praise the man's political wisdom, and still be sceptical
about his party's chances. It looks as if this sentence is intentional on Chisholm's criterion, with 'whatever will bring him
victory in the next election' as the intentional object. There is,
however, clearly no psychological element in it. 'Do' is precisely
the kind of verb which is not thought to be intentional. It
is significant that the sentence 'The Prime Minister will do
whatever he thinks will bring him victory in the next election'
has a different meaning. It is far less complimentary about the
Prime Minister's sagacity. Even if there was something which
would bring his party victory, the second sentence does not
suggest that the Prime Minister would necessarily do it.

[1] cf. Ryle, *The Concept of Mind*, p. 222.

Does the criterion of referential opacity fare any better? Is it either a necessary or a sufficient condition for intentionality? If it were sufficient, there would be plenty of sentences which would apparently be intentional even though they were far from being descriptions of psychological phenomena. For example, the prettiest village in England might also be the village with the worst parking problem. It is necessarily true that the prettiest village in England is the prettiest village in England. It does not follow that it is necessarily true that the prettiest village in England is the village with the worst parking problem.

Is the criterion necessary? We have seen that it is possible to recognize someone under one description and not under another. If I recognize a man, and fail to realize it is the mayor, I might deny having recognized the mayor. Yet in so far as I greeted him as an acquaintance, was it not true that I did recognize the mayor? Similarly if I know Mr. Smith and he is the mayor, it is true that I know the mayor whether I realize it or not. I can know someone without knowing that I know him. Clearly I would deny knowledge of the mayor in all sincerity, but if someone were to say of me 'He knows the mayor', that person would be quite right. On the other hand, if I know that Mr. Smith is ill, it by no means follows that I know that the mayor is ill. I could send my good wishes for Mr. Smith's recovery and then set out for an appointment with the mayor. I could recognize that Mr. Smith was the best man available for some task and deny that the mayor was. On this criterion therefore 'know' and 'recognize' appear to be intentional when followed by a propositional clause but not when they take a direct object. This seems a very surprising conclusion. If the purpose of these criteria is to distinguish psychological from non-psychological verbs, it seems very odd to find that in the case of 'know' and 'recognize' it all depends on what we know and what we recognize.

It might be objected that 'know' and 'recognize' are already suspect because they demand the existence of their object. I can however be angry at something which has not in fact happened or with someone who does not exist. I might be angry with Mr. Smith and deny that I was angry with the mayor, because of my ignorance that Smith is mayor. Would it be nevertheless correct for someone to say of me that I am angry with the mayor? If my anger reaches the point where I hit Smith, it is certainly true that I am hitting the mayor. Is it not also true that I am angry with the mayor? Am I not mistaken if I deny it? No one would dream of saying that although I hit the mayor I was not angry with *him*. 'I am angry with Smith' seems to be intentional, while 'He is angry with the mayor' is not. It seems hardly likely that the first refers to a psychological phenomenon and the second does not, when both sentences are descriptions of the same occurrence.

The same kind of consideration can be pressed even with such a central psychological verb as 'thinking'. I might think that Smith is incompetent and yet deny that I thought the mayor incompetent. It would still be true in some sense that I thought that the mayor was incompetent, even though to say so would be to go beyond my actual thoughts. It is significant that in this situation I cannot myself say, 'I think that the mayor is incompetent', while other people who know that Smith is mayor might say, 'He thinks that the mayor is incompetent'. According to the criterion of referential opacity the first sentence is intentional and the second is not. In other words, 'thinking' both is and is not a psychological verb. It could be retorted that the criterion does distinguish between what I actually think and a report of my thoughts which goes beyond them. It shows which is the genuine intentional object (i.e. what I actually think). However, according to Chisholm's second criterion (that the propositional clause is not implied to be true or false) both sentences are intentional.

Clashes of this sort further demonstrate that as a device for accurately distinguishing psychological from non-psychological phenomena the kind of grammatical criteria proposed by Chisholm and Miss Anscombe are worthless. They are neither necessary nor sufficient. Nevertheless they certainly point to interesting logical features of experiences which involve some sort of thought or awareness. It is important that we can think of something which does not exist, and that we can be aware of somebody under one description and not know any of the others which are true of him.

It is sometimes far from clear what the purpose is of finding out criteria for intentionality. Chisholm follows Brentano in hoping that they will distinguish the 'mental' from the 'physical'. Miss Anscombe pays less attention to this and seems to want to distinguish 'intentional objects' from other types of grammatical objects. As a result she is more interested in classifying the direct object in a sentence than the verb, and the classification appears to become an end in itself. Furthermore it is sometimes difficult to decide what exactly the intentional object is. If I say, 'I am angry with Smith for insulting me', what is the object, Smith, the insult, or Smith and the insult? If I said I was angry with Smith without giving a reason, presumably Smith would be regarded as the 'object' all on his own. If I said I was angry about the insult, presumably that would be an object on its own. If either Smith or the insult could be an object, it might appear that when I claim to be angry with Smith because of the insult, I am specifying two objects. On the other hand, I am not angry twice over, once with Smith and once about the insult, so perhaps there is only one object. We are given no way of deciding.

The whole course of the controversy about 'intentional objects' has made it obvious that by 'object' was meant something on the model of 'Socrates' in 'I am thinking about Socrates'. Such an object is easily identifiable and uncomplicated. However, many candidates for the title 'intentional object' are not at all like that. In the past few pages we have mentioned objects such as 'that the Queen of the United Kingdom is also Queen of Australia'. If it were suggested that the Queen is the object, then who, real or imagined, is the object in the sentence, 'I hope that someone will give the country the lead it needs'? Once again, we meet the question how it can be decided what the intentional object is. Is it, in the first example, 'the Queen' or the whole proposition? If we are led by the imagery of 'aiming at' suggested by the Latin word *intendo* (the root of 'intentional') we might think that the Queen was the 'object' on whom our thoughts were directed. On the other hand, if we wish to emphasize that an intentional object is a type of grammatical object, we might incline to saying that the whole clause was the object. This approach could bring us some very complicated objects, if, for instance, the 'object' of my thought is what I am thinking at a particular moment. I might be thinking that certain technical measures might provide a limited answer to the underlying weakness of the economy. Miss Anscombe provides examples of 'intentional' verbs by comparing 'thinking' and 'worshipping' with 'shooting at' or 'aiming'.[1] 'Worshipping' fits more closely into the pattern than 'thinking', but the very fact that Miss Ancombe uses this particular comparison is instructive. She has assumed what an 'object' is without really examining the term. Just as we aim an arrow or a gun at a stag, and worship a god, so she concludes that we must think about some simple object of the same type.

It is very easy to talk about an emotion being directed at an object, but this metaphor does make certain unjustifiable assumptions about what kind of thing the object is. We can aim a shot at a target, but what is my fear directed at when I am afraid that the Government will be impetuous—the Government, its impetuosity or the whole proposition? Nevertheless, however dubious the concept of an intentional object is, there is still a distinction to be made between the cause of fear and what we are afraid of. To talk of an emotion being 'object-directed' may very well be to use misleading imagery, but it must be a conceptual truth that every emotion involves an awareness of something beyond itself. I can never be angry without being angry at something, and I must know what this is. Normally, what makes me angry is what I am angry about. It is possible to be angry because of one's indigestion, without being angry *at* my indigestion, and it is this distinction which must be sustained. The kind of criteria which we have examined will clearly not be any use in pointing out any 'intentional object'. The key must rather lie in the fact that if I am angry at my indigestion, I must believe I have indigestion. I must always be able to answer the question 'What are you angry about?' On the other hand, if the indigestion is merely the cause of my anger about something else, I may be in complete ignorance of it.

I can be aware of many things, when in the grip of an emotion, which are not the 'object' (for want of a better word)

[1] 'The Intentionality of Sensation', *Analytical Philosophy*, ed. Butler, (second series), p. 167.

of the emotion. I may even realize that what I am angry at is not the cause of my anger. The fact that I know I have indigestion does not make it the 'object' of my anger. This is shown by the fact that if I forget the latter or realize that the true situation is not as I thought, my emotion will be dissipated. It will not help at all to dampen my emotion if I forget my indigestion. The presence of an emotion depends on our viewing the situation in a particular way. If we stop thinking about it, or come to see it in a different light (if, for example, we see that something wasn't really an insult), our emotion will leave us. Even in the case of such things as irrational fears, there must be a sense in which we believe that something is threatening us, and react to the situation accordingly, even if at the same time we recognize that there is no adequate reason for our apprehension. Until our 'belief' can be removed our fear will remain. Indeed it could be said that the thought of what we see as a threat *is* the fear, whether it is particularly emotional or not. For this reason it is true of fear that the more dangerous we conceive something as being, the more afraid we are, and the more we give way to fear, the more we become obsessed with the thought of danger.

The other emotions show similar patterns. A mother might become anxious because her child is late home. We only say that she is *anxious* because she has realized the child has been delayed *and* views it with concern. However, just as she becomes more anxious as she thinks about it more, her anxiety makes her think more about the child. Her thoughts and her anxiety are not logically distinct. She could not have had the same thoughts without being anxious, because to think about a child's lateness and to be concerned about it, to view it as an ominous sign, is to be anxious. In other words, mere awareness of something can be dispassionate and is not a sufficient vehicle for emotion. It is necessary to see it in a particular light.

If we ask whether pain is like the emotions in so far as it demands an 'object', we are at least asking whether we have to be aware of anything besides the sensation to be in pain. Clearly we do not need to know what is causing our pain in order to know whether we are feeling pain or not. When we feel pain, do we have to be aware of something else? Must we be viewing a situation in a particular way? When we suffer mental pain or distress, we do not just feel something. We must be thinking of some situation we dislike. When we feel physical pain, however, we do not have to be aware of anything besides the sensation. If we forget what is distressing us, our distress will go. Apart from the sensation, there is nothing which we can try to forget when we are in physical pain. A sensation does not require the thought of anything else. As a result, argument cannot affect the sensations I feel. Unlike emotion they do not depend on beliefs which can be changed.

II

'PAIN-QUALITY'

1. *Unpleasant Sensations and Pains*

AN 'aspect theorist' like Marshall, who was quoted at the beginning of Chapter I, insisted that pleasure and pain 'are grasped mentally very much as other qualities of a general character are grasped'. He continued: 'We recognize that a content has pleasure-pain quality, then, much as we recognize that a content has intensity.' This is to treat all pleasure and pain on the model of sensations. It is not surprising that the aspect theory worked better with sensations, which can have specific qualities and be of a certain intensity, than with mental pain. Marshall himself reluctantly admitted that there are states of mind in which the pleasure-pain quality is the only thing we can grasp. One example he gives is 'the pain one feels when thinking of a dear friend who lies dangerously ill far away'.

The aspect theory treated both mental and physical pain alike but analysed both in a way more suited to physical pain. An analysis of physical pain as 'an emotion of distress or displeasure at a sensation' tries to assimilate all pain to mental pain, with, as we have seen, all differences confined to the types of 'object' the emotion takes. We can expect, therefore, that it will be at its strongest where the aspect theory fails, but that it may get into difficulties itself where the aspect theory is at its strongest.

To talk of a 'pain-quality' in connection with sensations does explain why it is that pain sensations are so distinctive. Not only do they press themselves on our attention, but we usually have no difficulty in deciding whether what we feel is a pain or not. It is not just that we dislike a pain or want to be rid of it. It seems to have a distinct 'feel' about it, just as the colour 'red' has a distinct 'look' about it. If asked to explain the meaning of 'red' to someone, we are reduced to pointing out a succession of different red things—a pillar-box, a London Transport bus and so on—and to hoping that our pupil will latch on to what it is that the different objects have in common. If he does, he will be able to name as 'red' new red objects of different shapes and sizes, as he sees them. Much the same kind of thing has to happen with pain. If someone wanted to know what we meant by pain, we would eventually be forced to inflict different kinds of pain on him—kick him, prick him with a pin and so on—and hope that he would see that the different sensations he felt did have something in common. We would also have to ensure that he could differentiate between these and unpleasant sensations (of pressure etc.) which were not pains. If he did he would henceforth be able to use the word in other situations where he felt a similar 'quality'. His behaviour would of course usually have to be appropriate to a man in pain, or else we might begin to wonder if he could really feel pain or was insensitive to it. He would, too, be expected to use the word in typical pain-producing contexts, just as the man being taught the meaning of 'red' would be expected to use the word when confronted with such things as pillar-boxes. Otherwise we would not be convinced that they had really understood the meaning of the words.

Wittgenstein's concern that a sincere avowal of pain should leave no possibility of error leads him to talk of someone who had been taught the concept—'perhaps by means of gestures or pricking him with a pin'.[1] 'If he now said, for example,' Wittgenstein continues, ' "Oh, I know what 'pain' means; what I don't know is whether *this*, that I have now, is pain"— we should merely shake our heads and be forced to regard his words as a queer reaction which we have no idea what to do with.' Even if one wants to keep the incorrigibility of avowals inviolate, this is far too extreme a position, as it seems to deny the possibility of ever questioning the extension of any concept. The same argument would tell against someone who said, 'Oh, I know what "mammal" means; what I don't know is whether this whale is a mammal.' Such a person would surely be showing a natural bewilderment rather than 'a queer reaction we have no idea what to do with'. All we have to do

[1] *Philosophical Investigations*, § 288.

is to satisfy him that, despite appearances, whales do meet the requirements of the definition of mammals. Similarly someone who wondered whether 'this electric shock I'm feeling is pain' would be merely worrying over a very real problem about how far the concept of pain extends. There is no question of being mistaken about the sensation in this context, or of taking it 'for something other than what it is'. That kind of problem is completely separate from this issue, which is only incidentally concerned with the sensation the person is at that moment having. Implicit in his bewilderment is the conceptual question as to whether electric shocks in general can be classified as pains.

In fact the analysis of pain as 'distress at a sensation' would have the effect of classifying electric shocks, and other sensations which are generally unpleasant, as pains. There are, however, certain types of sensations, which are extremely distressing and yet are not called 'pains'. We can wind a piece of string around our finger, endure progressively greater discomfort, and finally find it intolerable. Yet we would be disinclined to call the localized and distinctly unpleasant sensation a 'pain'. Electric shocks seem to come into this category. Although they are usually disliked, they are often not regarded as 'painful'. It is also significant that some Chinese tortures (such as tickling fettered feet) involved no physical pain.

H. Head[1] conducted some very interesting experiments which threw light on this point and led to his distinction between the 'sensory quality' of pain and the 'feeling-tone' of 'discomfort' which usually accompanied it. He was particularly concerned with the effect of an electric current on a leg which was 'totally insensitive to painful stimulation of all kinds, in consequence of an intramedullary lesion'. He found that 'so long as tactile sensibility remains perfect (the patient) will complain bitterly of the discomfort caused by this form of stimulation'. Experiments with two patients 'showed that the movement of withdrawal seemed to be almost as violent when a current of known strength was applied to the analgesic as to the normal leg'. Head reports that one patient 'said the sensation produced was a "kind of exaggerated tickling more

[1] *Studies in Neurology*, ii. 405.

unpleasant than pain". Both these patients were firm in their assertions that the sensation was not painful; and yet an observer watching their behaviour would suppose they were undergoing intolerable pain.'

Situations like these seem to show that the emotional component of pain can be combined with some types of sensations and yet neither the resulting complex nor the 'bare sensation' (if such a thing be possible) be called 'pain'.

What of the theory that 'pain' should be analysed as 'distress at certain types of distinctive bodily sensations' and that cutting, throbbing and burning sensations can be given as examples? Broad[1] puts forward a view of this kind, when he distinguishes pains from other unpleasant experiences by saying:

There are certain qualities which are sensibly manifested mainly in intra-somatic sensation, e.g. throbbingness, burningness, stabbingness, etc. For most people these qualities are strongly unpleasant making even when they are manifested with only slight intensity. What we call 'a pain' is an unpleasant experience which owes its unpleasantness to the fact that in it one of these qualities is sensibly manifested.

However, what of those (and it is implied that there are some) who do not find one of 'these qualities' unpleasant—perhaps because of the low intensity of the sensation? Broad would presumably not allow their sensation to be called 'a pain'. The last sentence of the quotation suggests that, taken separately, the unpleasantness of a sensation and one of 'these qualities' are to be regarded as necessary but not sufficient conditions for the attribution of pain. How are we to decide what 'these qualities' are? By his inclusion of 'et cetera' after his three examples, Broad indicates that there are a lot of other similar types of sensation. There are, for instance, pricking, shooting, gnawing, bursting and stinging sensations, to mention a few more adjectives. As these words are often coupled with 'pain' it is reasonable to suppose that 'for most people these qualities are strongly unpleasant making'. Is a gnawing sensation of hunger to be called a pain? Presumably it must depend on how unpleasant it is. It is a matter of

[1] *Examination of McTaggart's Philosophy*, ii, pt. i, 130.

common experience that some pricking sensations are not unpleasant. Presumably then they cannot be regarded as pains.
Even Broad's original 'qualities' regularly appear with neutral
sensations. Not all throbbing sensations are pains (what of the
throb of a heart-beat?) whilst a burning sensation in my throat
is different from a sore throat (and even that is not called a
'pain in the throat' though we do talk of it 'hurting to swallow').

Broad is on rather firmer ground with 'stabbing sensations'.
Most, if not all, such sensations do happen to be pains, but this
is surely because of the dramatic imagery employed. To talk of
something stabbing one is to suggest something that cannot
be ignored, something that demands an emotional reaction
from us. The analogy must surely be this way round, with the
pain being compared to other things that stab us. Many
philosophers, however, have not understood it in this way.
Ryle,[1] for example, suggests: 'When a sufferer describes a
pain as a stabbing, a grinding or a burning pain, though he
does not necessarily think that his pain is given to him by a
stiletto, a drill or an ember, still he says what sort of a pain it
is by likening it to the sort of pain that would be given to
anyone by such instruments.' However if we have never been
stabbed—and most people have not—how could we possibly
know what sort of pain is caused by stabbing? The same kind
of objection applies to the other analogies. Can we be sure
that 'burning pains' are in fact the kind of pains we get when
burnt? Surely we can use and understand such imagery before
we have been burnt ourselves? The case of shooting pains
provides an obvious counter-example to Ryle's explanation.
They are certainly not the kinds of pain one would feel when
shot. The comparison is rather between such a pain and, say, a
shooting star, the predominant idea being that of the rapid
motion of the pain and of the star. Pricking pains, on the other
hand, are very similar to the pains caused by pricking. Maybe
the truth is that, although all the imagery we use to describe
our pains has to be drawn from the external world (so as to
establish communication between ourselves and others), they
are not all drawn in the same way. Just because a pricking
pain may be like a pain caused by pricking, it does not follow
that a shooting pain is like a pain caused by shooting.

[1] *Concept of Mind*, p. 203.

To return to Broad's theory, it looks as if our decision as to whether a pricking sensation, for example, is a pain must depend on whether it is unpleasant. Broad's 'et cetera' after his examples suggests that any non-perceptual bodily sensation can be a candidate for being called a pain. The kind of experience he wants to rule out is indicated by his assertion that 'not all experiences which are highly unpleasant are pains. Thus the experiences of smelling sulphuretted hydrogen or tasting castor-oil are extremely unpleasant to most people but they are not counted as pains.' Bodily sensations are certainly involved in these cases of perception, and the examples certainly show that there are extremely unpleasant sensations which cannot be called pains. Is Broad justified in concluding that this is because the qualities of 'throbbingness, burningness, stabbingness, etc.', are absent? After all, a very bright light is not only unpleasant but positively painful to look at. Although there may be a connection here with bodily injury, there are certainly no throbbing sensations or anything similar. Perhaps Broad's examples of unpleasant sensations of taste and smell which are not pains are merely witnesses against his own theory. As we have seen, this all too often reduces, in fact if not in intention, to an equation of pain and unpleasantness.

The fundamental objection to Broad's whole approach is that it puts the cart before the horse. It suggests that we classify sensations as shooting sensations, or throbbing sensations, before we classify them as pains. In fact, however, it seems natural to call a sensation a 'pain' before we search around for analogies with which to describe it. There is not a genus of 'shooting sensations' with a sub-class of those we especially dislike (i.e. pains). There is rather a genus of pains, and an analogy with shooting stars somehow seems appropriate for a type of pain within that genus. This is reasonable, as it is far more important to us that the sensation is a pain than that it is, say, a stinging kind of sensation. The sensation of pain is a sign of the malfunctioning of some part of the body, and this is obviously of vital concern. A description of the type of pain may be useful to the doctor in his diagnosis, but we have to be prompted to go to the doctor first. The insistent quality of pain is well equipped to make us do this.

3

Does this quality consist in anything more than the unpleasantness of pain, in anything other than the fact that we do dislike certain sensations? We have already seen the attraction of thinking of a pain-quality and the inadequacy of theories that dismiss the whole idea. Linguistic considerations offer further evidence of this. If asked why we disliked a certain thing, to say that it was because it was unpleasant is really to give no answer. It tells us nothing new and the questioner would naturally be prompted to ask in what way it was unpleasant. If we replied that it was because it was hurting us, because it was painful, or because it was giving us a pain (phrases that are roughly synonymous), the questioner would be satisfied. We would have given him fresh information. If it were objected that the only new knowledge he had was that it was a sensation that we disliked, we could compare the answers to the question 'Why do you dislike that sensation?'. To be told that it is because it is unpleasant is to have the dislike of the sensation merely reaffirmed. The answer 'Because it hurts' or 'Because it's painful' not only rules out many unpleasant types of sensation but explains why we dislike that sensation. Similarly the statement that a sensation 'is unpleasant, but isn't painful' is not a contradiction. It tells us that the sensation may be disliked, but nevertheless does not have that distinctive and insistent quality which marks off pain from other sensations. It is however as impossible to describe what the quality of pain is as it is to describe any other unanalysable quality like redness.

2. *Pain-Quality*

The concept of a 'pain-quality' becomes necessary when it is realized that pains are not defined as merely unpleasant sensations. It cannot be the case that we just group some sensations together without any basis for doing so. We must be able to explain our ability to cope with completely new types of sensations. We do not have to think of our reaction to the sensation or the context in which it occurs before saying whether they are new types of *pain* or not. There is clearly something about a sensation in itself which prompts us to declare that it is a pain, and if this element is absent, we deny that the sensation is to be classed as a pain. It is perhaps important to stress that this is not an instance of the *unum nomen, unum nominatum* fallacy. We are not assuming that because there is one name 'pain' it must name one thing. We shall later argue that 'pleasure' does *not* name a sensation. 'Pain', however, is used to refer to *some* types of sensation which are generally unpleasant, and not to others. If we do not use it in a completely arbitrary manner, the reason must be that it refers only to one class of sensation.

There must be some similarity between various sensations which is sufficiently marked to induce us to group the sensations together as the same kind of sensation and give the same name to them all. It is this for which we have coined the term 'pain-quality'. It is an important factor in the distinctions we make between different kinds of bodily sensations. Without the notion of a pain-quality we would be able to make nothing of the distinction which people often want to make[1] between a pricking sensation and a pricking pain, or a stinging sensation and a stinging pain. Pricking pains are different from unpleasant pricking sensations, so it is irrelevant whether we dislike the sensation. Without the notion of a pain-quality it would be utterly mysterious why we should gain more information about a sensation if told that it was painful than if we merely heard that it was unpleasant. The notion explains why we can tell people that we have a pain if we are asked what kind of sensation we feel. If the word 'pain' does not refer to a special class of sensation, this answer would be curiously inappropriate. As it is, the word clearly marks off sensations from tingles, tickles, throbs and a host of other sensations which we are quite certain are not pains.

We have compared 'pain-quality' to red, but it can be objected that there are many different kinds of pain. Might it not be more enlightening to compare it with colour? There need then be no misleading implication that every pain feels exactly the same. Plato makes Socrates take a similar line in the *Philebus*[2] in response to an assertion that pleasures cannot be different in kind from each other, since that would be to make something different from itself. Socrates points out that one colour can differ from another and that black is the

---

[1] See Chapter VIII *init.*
[2] *Philebus* 12E.

opposite of white even though both are still called colours.
Cannot we say that just as there is a spectrum of colours there
is also a spectrum of pains? 'Colour', however, is an all-
embracing term in a way in which 'pain' is not. There are
sensations which are not pains, just as there are other colours
which can be contrasted with red. We can say that something
is not red but orange, and we can say that something is not a
pain but a pricking sensation. There are, however, no 'non-
colours' to contrast with colours. Pains and tingles can be
subsumed under the concept of sensation, and orange and red
under the concept of colour, but it is not so easy to group
colour with anything else under a further concept.

Pain should be compared with a colour rather than with
colour in general. This need not suggest that the concept of
pain-quality implies that all pains feel exactly the same any
more than that the concept of red implies that there are not
different shades of red. We recognize that vermilion, scarlet
and crimson have a place within the concept of red, and it
would be reasonable to suppose that there may be different
kinds of pain which are nevertheless related in an important
way. The term 'pain-quality' is not intended to rule this out.
It might even be more correct to think of a range or spectrum
of pain-qualities. 'Pain-quality', however, does indicate that
pains are related in the same respect, namely in the way that
they feel. Pains are not classified as the same kind of sensation
because of our reaction to them, as we shall see that itches are.
They are not grouped together because of their duration or
location. A 'twinge' conceptually must only last for a brief
period of time, whereas pains can last for a moment or a very
long time. A 'headache' could not be anywhere but in our
head. Even if we felt exactly the same kind of sensation elsewhere it would not be a 'headache'. Pains, on the other hand,
can clearly be felt anywhere and still be pains. Intensity is
also irrelevant to the concept of pain. Pains can be either mild
or intense in a way that 'agony' cannot.

The fact that pains are similar *in the same respect* indicates
that it might be misleading to talk in terms of a 'family resemblance' between them. Wittgenstein thought that there
was no one respect in which games were similar.[1] Instead, he

---

[1] *Philosophical Investigations*, § 66.

said, 'we see a complicated network of similarities overlapping and criss-crossing: sometimes overall similarities, sometimes similarities of detail'. He called these 'family resemblances', because he saw that resemblances between different members of a family 'overlap and criss-cross in the same way'. Wittgenstein mentions such things as build, features, colour of eyes, gait and temperament. Clearly a family could have a set of marked characteristics without any one characteristic being shared by all the members of a family. A Churchill could look like one without having a Churchill nose. An activity can be clearly a game without involving a ball. A sensation cannot be a pain without the one element of 'pain-quality'. It changes and becomes a different sort of sensation with a different name if it either gains or loses this one feature. All other points about a sensation are irrelevant to the question whether it is a pain. It is enough for a sensation to feel like a pain to be a pain. In this respect, too, any analogy with games or families breaks down. It is not enough to look like a Churchill in order to be a Churchill, and there is an important distinction between being like a game and being a game. Something may be fun and have a lot in common with games, but if it has a serious purpose it is incorrect, or perhaps cynical, to call it a game. The fact that doing philosophy can be fun not does make it a game. Surf-riding is fun and in addition has no particularly serious purpose, but it is still not a game.

The force of talking about a *quality* of pain comes from the fact that pain is a kind of sensation, and it is always possible to identify a sensation without paying regard to its quality (or what kind it is). It is enough for me to locate it. I can then identify it by its position and talk, for instance, of 'the sensation in my leg'. It is this which enables us to say a particular sensation has changed into a pain. It is logically possible to identify what has pain-quality without knowing it has the quality. There is a logical distinction, although perhaps not a temporal one, between identifying the sensation and recognizing its quality. It is logically possible to glimpse a chair and not notice its colour. In the same way we might feel a twinge and not notice whether it was a twinge of pain or not. The point is not merely that we would be uncertain whether to call it a pain, but that we genuinely did not notice what kind

of twinge it was. It came and went too quickly. We might
know that we had felt something in our leg, and that would be
all.

It is sometimes difficult to decide whether a particular
object is red or, say, purple. We might compromise and say
finally that it was purplish red. Clearly the same difficulty
sometimes arises with pain. Electric shocks are generally
found to be unpleasant, but there might be hesitation as to
whether they were *pains*. The disagreement could arise from
the way they feel, and not from any prejudice that unpleasant
sensations must be pains. Any hesitation would suggest that
electric shocks are to be placed at the boundaries of pain.
What if there was disagreement between people who had
previously shown that they had a full grasp of the concept of
pain, and one person firmly asserted that an electric shock
produced pain, while someone else denied it? It could be that
electric shocks did not have uniform effects. They might indeed cause pain in some people and not in others. If, however,
someone said firmly that an object (which was in fact purplish
red) was simply red, what would our attitude be? Would we
accuse him of illegitimately extending the concept of red?
There are two possibilities. The object may look red to him,
when most others agree that it is purplish red. In other words,
he may not be able to distinguish the colour from that of a
pillar-box, whereas others wish to discriminate between the
two. On the other hand, he may admit that the colour looks
very different from what he accepts are central cases of red,
but still wishes to say it is red. The first possibility is an instance of an abnormality in his sight. The second suggests a
divergence from normal opinions about the boundaries of the
concept. He wishes to call a certain thing 'red' when the others
do not. The conclusion must be that he is mistaken in ignoring
distinctions which everyone else thinks important, although his
inclination to use the word 'red' might suggest that we are
dealing with a fairly border-line case.

How are disagreements about the boundary of the concept of
pain to be resolved? It is possible that two people who dis-
agreed about whether the sensation produced by an electric
shock was a pain or not are disagreeing about the boundaries
of the concept of pain. Might not the boundaries be very

unclear? Indeed, may not different languages put them in different places? As with a disagreement over whether something looks red, it is important to distinguish between a definite abnormality in a person feeling a sensation and a conceptual disagreement about how to classify it. I might say that electric shocks produced sensations very similar to central cases of pain, or I might agree that it felt significantly different but not different enough to refuse to call it a pain. Others might consider that in their case the difference was marked enough to make it a completely different kind of sensation. The situation, of course, is more complicated than in the case of a disagreement over colour. We can all argue about the colour of the same object, but we cannot all have numerically the same sensation. Because we cannot check whether the way people describe their sensations is accurate, the notion of accuracy or inaccuracy can have no place here. It is, however, vitally important that before any discussion starts we know we can rely on what someone says. For this reason, any disagreement about whether to call a sensation occurring in a certain context 'pain' is only interesting and significant if the disputants have fully learned the concept of pain. We shall deal more fully with the importance of this later. It is reasonable to assume that disagreements about whether a sensation is a pain would not be the result of any great conviction on either side. They would rather be a sign that one was on the boundaries of the concept of pain, and no definite decision might be able to be given. People with normal sight and a knowledge of colour concepts do not disagree violently over whether a purplish red is to be called 'red' or not. They realize that such an argument would merely oversimplify the position.

One line of thought must be resisted. There may be doubt and hesitation about the boundaries of the concept of pain. It does *not* follow that there must be doubt and hesitation in every case of pain. Just because we are reluctant to call some buses 'red' which only have a red tinge in their colouring, it does not follow that, if we have a full grasp of the concept of red, we should have any doubt at all over the question whether an ordinary London Transport bus in normal light looks red or not. Indeed, if we did hesitate, this would suggest that we did not know the meaning of 'red' (or that there was something wrong with our eyes). Trouble with boundary-cases of pain is equally irrelevant to central cases. We must not assume that because hesitation about the extension of the concept is sometimes in order it is always in order. Although we should sometimes be wary about someone's claim that a sensation is a pain, it would be ludicrous for us always to be wary. If someone who is conceptually well-educated is writhing in apparent agony after a wound and complains of pain at the site of the wound, it is out of order for us (unless there are very special and peculiar circumstances) to ask if he may not be extending the concept of pain illegitimately. Similarly if someone says that he has a sensation exactly like the sensations he has always called 'pain', but that this time strangely enough he does not dislike it, the only reason to suppose that he is extending the concept in calling this sensation 'pain' is the strangeness of a pain which is not disliked. That, however, is a different question from the one concerning the difficulty which may arise in boundary-cases when classifying a sensation according to its quality. If the sensation is 'exactly like' those occurring in obvious cases of pain, it is pain. The trouble arises in cases where it is agreed to be rather different. It is significant that in the cases which we shall be discussing, where people talk of 'pain' in situations where they do not dislike it, they are not talking of new kinds of sensations, or sensations which just have *something* in common with normal pains. They are describing ordinary pains with normal causes and often say that the sensation is exactly the same as one they normally find unpleasant. Indeed in experiments to measure the threshold of pain, the subjects say that they recognize a sensation as pain and later come to dislike what they say is the same sensation.[1]

How could one be sure that the sensation is the same each time? Might someone only think it was the same because his memory was mistaken? Does not the picture of someone recognizing a sensation as being 'pain again' immediately raise the possibility that his purported recognition was in fact no recognition at all? If I say that a sensation has what we have termed 'pain-quality' and am inclined to give it the name 'pain', what I say is unverifiable. This might suggest that we can never be sure that the pain-quality does not constantly

[1] See Chapter VIII *init.*

change, and that our memory does not constantly deceive us. This is the kind of argument employed by Wittgenstein in the *Philosophical Investigations* to show that there is no place in concepts, which by their very nature are public, for 'private objects' which in principle are available only to one person. He says[1]:

'Imagine a person whose memory could not retain what the word "pain" meant so that he constantly called different things by that name—but nevertheless used the word in a way fitting in with the usual symptoms and presuppositions of pain'—in short he uses it as we all do. Here I should like to say: a wheel that can be turned though nothing else moves with it is not part of the mechanism.

It will be our contention in subsequent chapters that to ignore the importance for the concept of pain of the way the sensation feels is in fact to rule out too many ways in which people do use the word 'pain'. The difference between the concept of pain as it is and the concept of pain without the element of 'pain-quality' is quite considerable. In other words, whatever Wittgenstein might say, 'pain-quality' is one of our normal presuppositions about pain. If we ignore this, we are left with no way of explaining why we call some unpleasant sensations 'pains' and not others. 'Pain' has then to come to mean 'unpleasant sensation'. Without the concept of pain-quality we can make no distinction between the reporting of a pain in abnormal circumstances (when, for instance, it is not disliked) and the misreporting of pain. Clearly, however, the distinction might be of vital importance. Pains usually have medical significance. Indeed, they are almost invariably a sign of the malfunctioning of a part of the body. A doctor would be more concerned with a pain which occurs in an abnormal situation than with a tingle which, perhaps as a result of a basic ignorance about the concept, was misreported as pain. His only problem will be how to distinguish the two in practice.

Wittgenstein's views on the impossibility of a 'private language' composed of words which can only be known to the person speaking depend on beliefs about the nature of concepts (i.e. what it is for a general word or an expression to have

[1] § 271.

meaning). A proper consideration of his position would take us far away from the particular problems of the concept of pain. However, his emphasis on the difficulties which ensue if we treat sensations on the model of public objects and allow the possibility of error in someone's sincere report of them is clearly relevant. Once people have learnt the concept of pain, no sense can be given to the question whether their sensation really has 'pain-quality' even though they say it is a pain. We have no way of correcting them, and a position of sceptical doubt is clearly out of place.

3. *The Duality of Pain*

It might be suggested that painfulness is just an extreme form of unpleasantness. In that case only extremely unpleasant sensations would be pains. There would be no need for only mildly unpleasant ones to be regarded as such. This was the view held by Marshall and the aspect theorists. However, degrees of unpleasantness seem irrelevant to the assessment of whether a sensation is a pain or not. Some sensations such as those of nausea are extremely disagreeable, and they are not pains. We must remember Head's patient who talked of 'a kind of exaggerated tickling more unpleasant than pain'. Surely this ought not to be ruled out *a priori* as being self-contradictory? On the other side, we must take account of the fact that sensations which are universally called 'pains' can be mildly unpleasant and distracting. Just because a pain in my finger is very slight this does not mean that it is not a pain.

Something of the aspect theory's insistence that pain is just an extreme form of displeasure seems to be unconsciously echoed by Armstrong. He claims[1]: 'The concept of physical pain is a portmanteau-concept: it involves *both* the having of a certain sort of bodily sense-impression, *and* the taking up of a certain attitude to the impression. The *painfulness* of the sense-impression is therefore a *relational* property of the impression, in just the same way that the painfulness of a scene is a relational property of the scene.' Armstrong goes on from this to conclude with the extraordinary remark that 'we call physical pain "pain" simply because the having of these impressions of bodily disturbance is normally the most painful

---

[1] *Bodily Sensations*, p. 107.

thing in human life'. As Armstrong is obviously using painful as a synonym of 'unpleasant' this is exactly the theory we dealt with in the last paragraph. There is, however, something very odd about the way Armstrong expresses it. Something that is painful must surely be something that affords us pain (whether pain is thought of as a sensation with a particular quality or as an emotion like distress). The concept of pain must logically be prior to that of 'being painful', whereas Armstrong seems to assume that the reverse is true.

Is Armstrong right in his more general point? Is the concept of physical pain a 'portmanteau-concept'? We have seen that when we talk of such pain, we are talking of a sensation with a particular quality. We have seen that the genus of what we call pain sensations—stabbing pains, shooting pains, burning pains and the rest—have got something in common other than that we usually dislike them. On the other hand the having of these sensations which we have no hesitation in just calling 'pains' does not constitute the whole experience of pain. The connection between 'physical' and 'mental' pain does not lie in the presence of these sensations, but in the emotional component which is usually a part of the experience of physical pain. It was suggested earlier that mental and physical pain each involved the same emotion (of pain or distress) but were differentiated by the type of 'object' they took. With 'mental pain' the distinction between emotion and 'object' is far more clear-cut than in a normal experience of 'physical pain'. The distress we feel at a bereavement is a very different kind of thing from the bereavement, which we certainly do not feel. A sensation of pain, on the other hand, is not so very different from the distress we feel at it. Both are experiences of a person, and it is reasonable to suppose that if both occur simultaneously, there will be no clear boundary between one and the other. This has led many to assume that there is only one experience when one is in pain, and this brings us to the paradox that pain seems to be both a sensation and an emotion. It is a sensation in so far as it can be localized and has its origin in a stimulus, and it is an emotion in so far as it disturbs one and makes one think of it as bad in some way. The paradox is immediately removed if the two strands are separated, and it is realized that the usual experience of pain involves both a sensation and an emotion directed at it.

Brentano saw this distinction. He realized, however, that it is very easy for the feeling of pain to swamp all other feelings and sensations. As he says[1], 'If someone is cut, then for the most part he has no further perception of touch: if he is burned no further perception of heat: but pain alone seems to be present in the one case and the other.' In the same way he thought that 'feelings' (or emotions) and 'sensations of feeling' (i.e. pleasure and pain) became regarded as a unity. He says[2]:

The object to which a feeling refers is not always an external object. Even when I hear a harmonious chord, the pleasure which I feel is not really a pleasure in the sound, but a pleasure in the hearing of it. Indeed one might not be mistaken in saying that it even refers to itself in a certain way and, therefore, that what Hamilton asserts, namely that the feeling is 'fused into one' with its object, *does* occur more or less.

Brentano goes on to point out that 'every fusion is a unification of several things', and there is still 'a certain duality in the unity'. It is not necessary to agree with Brentano that the emotional component of pain itself must always involve 'feelings', in order to assent to his main point that the distinction between the emotion and the sensation can become very blurred. Indeed Wittgenstein was able to deny that the two could in principle be distinguished, and could refer to pain-behaviour, which could be taken to be the behavioural manifestation of distress, as 'the expressions of the sensation'. It is significant that the word 'expression' has to be understood in a technical sense, as, although we talk of 'expressing our emotion', we never talk of 'expressing our sensation'.

Brentano claims that one reason for our confusion of the 'feeling' of pain and the 'sensation of feeling' is[3] 'that the quality on which the feelings ensues, and the feeling itself, do not bear two distinct names. We call the physical phenomenon, which occurs along with the feeling of pain, itself pain in this case.' He thinks that this is because the quality and the

---

[1] 'The Distinction between Mental and Physical Phenomena', in *Realism and the Background of Phenomenology*, ed. Chisholm, p. 44.
[2] op. cit. p. 52.   [3] op. cit. p. 46.

emotion stand in a very close relationship to each other, and he compares the equivocation with our practice of calling both body and food healthy. In fact, although we talk of feeling pain at situations, and in those contexts use it as a synonym for distress, we do not use it to refer to the emotion involved in an experience of physical pain. It is significant that in this chapter, when the components of the pain experience have been mentioned, the word 'pain' has had to be reserved for the sensation, and 'distress' has had to be used for the emotion. We just do not talk of feeling pain as a sensation. The ambiguity in the word 'pain' does not lie there, but in the fact that it can refer both to the 'simple' sensation, and to the whole pain experience—the combined sensation and emotion. It is because 'pain' has this ambiguity that 'I do not dislike that pain' can seem like a straight contradiction. If 'pain' means 'a sensation with a particular quality and dislike of (or distress at) it' the phrase is self-contradictory. If 'pain' means just 'a sensation with a particular quality' the phrase is certainly logical enough and might even be true. We need a word for the experience of emotion and sensation combined, and also one to mark off the genus of sensation from other unpleasant sensations, which do not have the same quality. Unfortunately 'pain' has to do duty for both. The word 'painful' seems to be more closely attached to the whole experience. If I find that a sensation is 'painful', I am not just recognizing it as a sensation of a certain distinctive quality. I am admitting that I am distressed by it. The same tendency is evident with the phrase 'being in pain'. If I am 'in pain', it would seem logically odd for me to be content with my situation, as the words seem to refer to the whole of my present experience rather than just to a sensation.

If there is a 'certain duality' in the unity of the experience of pain, and if an ambiguity in the word 'pain' to some extent draws attention to this, we would expect that it would be logically possible for the different parts of the experience to occur separately. The emotion of distress does arise in other contexts, although of course it always has an 'object' of some kind. It is very similar to (and perhaps a synonym of) mental pain. What of the sensation of pain? It must be logically possible for that to be had by someone who is not distressed by it. We shall see in a later chapter that it is not only logically possible, but does actually happen.

4. *Discomfort*

Is the concept of pain unique, or can a similar treatment be given to that of discomfort? Can we distinguish between mental and physical discomfort merely by noting a difference in the 'objects' of the two? As usual, we must be careful not to be trapped by any misleading implications the term 'object' has. The 'object' of mental discomfort, for example, is typically a situation we find uncomfortable. Just as I can be distressed by someone's remarks, I can also feel discomfort at them. A situation I find uncomfortable, or feel discomfort at, is one from which I want to be extricated. I am not, however, affected as deeply by it as I would be if I were distressed. The situation may be non-existent, but as long as I believe I am in it, I will feel discomfort.

Is physical discomfort just finding a sensation uncomfortable instead of a situation? There is, of course, a difference between 'finding a sensation uncomfortable', and 'feeling uncomfortable at a sensation'. In the latter case, the sensation itself is not the 'object'. We are uneasy about its significance, but if that was subtracted, we would not mind the sensation. Philosophers disagree over what is to be included in the category of physical discomfort. A. R. White thinks that a pain is a discomfort. He[1] distinguishes between 'momentary feelings such as stabs of pain . . . and the continuous discomforts, such as pains in the back, the itching of a rash or a tickling in the throat, of which these momentary feelings are the occurrent manifestations'. White obviously makes the duration of the feeling the criterion for calling it a 'discomfort'. He contrasts 'discomfort' with 'stabs' and 'twinges'. It would certainly be odd to talk of a 'momentary discomfort', as typical discomforts are the results of a gradual process, and increase in intensity slowly. However there is also a clear distinction between pains as a class and discomforts as a class, which rules out all possibility of terming any pain a 'discomfort'. Although some discomforts may be worse than mild pains, discomfort is typically more tolerable than pain. It is significant that much

[1] *Attention*, p. 35.

of what we call 'discomfort', if increased in intensity, can be recognized as pain. The discomfort of cold can easily become the pain of extreme cold. It does not take much for the pinching of an uncomfortable shoe to increase it to pain.

D. M. Armstrong[1] places 'bodily discomforts' in a third category alongside aches and pains. He says: 'I think they are more like aches than pains, but are even more vaguely and indeterminately located than aches. They come into being and die away even more gradually, and, characteristically, are not so intense. There seems to be no sharp distinction between aches and bodily discomforts.' Certainly, discomforts do not elicit as marked a reaction as aches, which we usually dislike more. To say that 'I find this ache uncomfortable' would be too mild, and would suggest that what we felt was not really an ache. Armstrong says nothing of the most definite distinction between aches and discomforts, the difference in the quality of the sensation. This is hardly surprising, as it is his aim to do away with such phenomenal entities, and to 'give an account of bodily sensation in terms of the concepts involved in perception: no unique, irreducible concepts are required'.[2] Thus with aches and pains he says that 'it feels to us as if a disturbance were occurring in a certain part of our body', whereas with discomforts 'our bodily impression may be be of nothing more than "something-or-other going on in a certain place" or perhaps "something amiss at a certain place".' Even if, when we have a pain, the disturbance feels, as Armstrong admits, like one 'of stabbing or tearing or burning', the distinctive quality of pain has been analysed out of existence. Armstrong wishes to say[3] that 'aches may be described as a species of physical pain'. On his analysis, there is no reason why discomforts should not be regarded as another such species. On the other hand, if we suppose that aches possess 'pain-quality' and are differentiated from pain merely by such facts as that aches tend to have a less precise location and to be 'duller' that pain, there is a clear distinction between them and discomfort. A discomfort would be yet another example of an unpleasant sensation which we refuse to call pain.

If discomforts are distinct from aches in not possessing 'pain-quality', what is it that makes us class so many different

[1] *Bodily Sensations*, pp. 111–12.   [2] ibid. p. 127.   [3] p. 111.

sensations as discomfort? What have the pinching of a shoe, a tickle, an itch, feeling cold and so on, all got in common? Perhaps a case can be made out for a special discomfort-quality, on the model of the distinctive quality of pain. Just as we can go on picking out red things and refusing to pick out non-red things just by their 'look', we may be able to assert in certain situations that the sensation we now felt was one of discomfort and in others to deny that it was, just by its 'feel'. This would give a sense to the concept of discomfort-quality, just as we have given a sense to that of pain-quality. As long as we satisfied others by our use of the word in typically uncomfortable situations that we did understand its correct use, it would be logically possible for us to say of a sensation that it was one of discomfort, but that we didn't mind it, or didn't find it unpleasant.

It is analytically true that if we find a sensation or feeling uncomfortable, we dislike it and think it unpleasant though in a milder way than if we are feeling a pain. Thus if it is possible to recognize a discomfort merely from the 'feel' of the sensation, regardless of our attitude to it, 'discomfort' has been prised apart from 'uncomfortable'. In that case, it would be possible not to find a sensation uncomfortable which we recognize as being one of discomfort. Conversely it would be possible to find sensations uncomfortable which we refused to call 'discomforts'. Both conditions hold good with 'pain' and 'unpleasant'. We do not necessarily find all sensations unpleasant which we recognize as 'pains', and we do find unpleasant some sensations which we do not call 'pains'.

It is however obvious that in ordinary speech 'discomfort' and 'uncomfortable' can each be used to describe the same situation without any change in meaning. A man who 'feels discomfort' is uncomfortable and vice versa. We are not in the one case describing the kind of sensation he is feeling and in the other telling of his reaction to it. 'Discomfort' would anyway not be a very informative word, if it were used just to describe the quality of the sensation. We may find sensations uncomfortable, and possibly call them 'discomforts', but if asked to describe them, we would not be content with the word 'discomfort'. Just to say that 'I feel discomfort in my foot' tells no one anything except that my foot feels uncomfortable.

Whether I have 'pins and needles' in it, or whether it is hot, cold, or just feeling numb is left unsaid. All these feelings can be sources of discomfort and yet it seems implausible that they all share the same quality. Indeed they all have distinctive and separate qualities. It seems likely that we call them discomforts because we have the same attitude towards them, that we want to be rid of them. Feeling physical discomfort is just finding certain sensations and feelings uncomfortable. It is feeling uncomfortable. Mental and physical discomfort can thus only be distinguished by the different type of 'object' each has. In this they are similar to the emotion involved in mental and physical pain.

III

THE EMOTIONAL COMPONENT

1. *Emotion and Pain*

As we have seen, the emotion of distress is often involved in an experience of physical pain. When someone writhes in agony, it is obvious that he is as much in the grip of an emotion as if he were furiously angry or mortally afraid. Emotions are characteristically instances of excitement and disturbance. They often overwhelm us, so that we are no longer calm and collected, and we show this on our faces and in our behaviour. It is hardly surprising that many have wanted to class pain with the emotions if emotion is a usual constituent of pain, and if typical pain-behaviour is an expression, not of a sensation, but of an emotion which has pain as its 'object'.

It is certainly plausible to talk in terms of emotion when pain is prolonged and severe. Our distress in such cases cannot be doubted. What of mild or momentary pains? We would usually dislike them and be glad to be rid of them. Even with a very mild twinge of pain we would typically rather be without it than with it. Could we in that case be said to be experiencing an emotion? Distress with a momentary pain as its 'object' would itself last only as long as the pain did, and Wittgenstein is sometimes thought to have queried whether there could be momentary emotions. He claimed[1]: 'If a man's bodily expression of sorrow and of joy alternated, say, with the ticking of a clock, here we should not have the characteristic formation of the pattern of sorrow or of the pattern of joy.' He is concerned to emphasize[2] that the surroundings give emotions their importance, and that whereas sensations do not depend on the context in which they occur for their significance, emotions do. He thus allows for the possibility of feeling 'violent pain' for a second but is uneasy about feeling 'deep grief' for a second. Certainly the way in which emotions have 'objects' guarantees

[1] *Philosophical Investigations*, II. i.   [2] op. cit. § 583.

that they logically cannot occur in isolation. Joy must be joy at something, and sorrow must be sorrow at something. If a man's sorrowful appearance alternated with a joyful one at the ticking of a clock, there would *ex hypothesi* be no 'object' for either emotion, and if that were so neither emotion could be identified as such in the first place. A facial expression or a feeling may be very similar to those that are connected with a particular emotion, but unless they occur in an intelligible context we cannot say anything more than that. A frown may be a sign of sorrow, indignation or worry, or it may be just a frown, depending on the context in which it occurs.

Wittgenstein asks[1]: 'Could someone have a feeling of ardent love or hope for the space of one second—*no matter what* preceded or followed this second?' It would be impossible to say that the feeling was one of love or hope, divorced from its surroundings. If, however, the feeling was placed in a suitable context, it does not necessarily follow then that I would be unable to identify the emotion. Our hearts may leap with hope at the sight of a letter bearing important news, but the hope may last only for the time it takes to seize the letter and open it. Just because our hopes are so swiftly dashed, are we to say that what we experienced was not hope? The context is surely sufficient for it to be identified as such. Wittgenstein puts the words 'no matter what' in italics and these give a subtle emphasis to his question. He is asking whether one could have a momentary feeling of love or hope, *whatever* the context. There is another answer to this question besides the one Kenny assumes,[2] that one cannot have a momentary emotion at all. This is that one could have a momentary feeling of love or hope if the context is specific enough, and if there is an explanation why the emotion is only momentary.[3] Wittgenstein's underlying point, that an emotion cannot be identified by the feeling often accompanying it, remains true, If the 'object' itself lasts only for a second, if our view of the situation is rapidly changed, then it is logically necessary that the incipient emotion itself disappears. If we start claiming that because it was so short-lived it could not have been an emotion, we have to ask how long we have to experience an emotion before we recognize it as one. How long do we have to think of something in a spirit of pleasurable anticipation

[1] § 583.   [2] *Action, Emotion and Will*, p. 58.   [3] *Bodily Sensations*, p. 90.

before we can admit that we are hopeful? Faced with this question, we must admit that the duration of an emotion must often be irrelevant to our identification of it. We do not wait five minutes to see if we still view a situation as threatening before claiming that we are afraid.

Wittgenstein has no qualms about the possibility of saying that 'for a second he felt violent pain' and regards this as an example of a use of the concept of sensation. What, however, of the word 'violent'? This may well suggest some emotional accompaniment to the sensation. Violent pains are usually pains which distress us a great deal because of their intensity. If the pain was less than violent, could an emotion still be involved?

First, what is the connection between the intensity of a pain and our dislike of it? Armstrong[1] says: 'A violent pain is a pain that we have an intense desire to stop. . . . A mild pain we would rather like to stop.' Later[2] he says: 'Intensity, or severity, we have suggested, is to be analysed in terms of the strength of our dislike of having the feeling'. This rules out the conceptual possibility of only having a mild wish that a violent pain should stop, or of having an intense desire that a mild pain should stop. It also suggests that if we do not dislike a pain at all it has not any intensity. Armstrong himself[3] admits that 'it is a contingent fact that we like or dislike certain bodily sense impressions'. It is hard to see how he can reconcile this with his assertion that descriptions such as 'pricking' and 'stinging'[4] are partly descriptions of the intensity of a pain. He would have to maintain that although we may not dislike pain in some instances, the use of such words as 'pricking' and 'stinging' entails that we do dislike the sensation. The fact that it is possible to talk of pricking sensations and stinging sensations and to deny that they are pains, or that we dislike them, would suggest that 'pricking' and 'stinging' refer to a type of sensation rather than to its intensity. It is quite usual to talk of a stinging sensation increasing in intensity. If 'stinging' partly refers to intensity, we would expect that our description of the sensation would change, as its intensity changed. Armstrong maintains that 'a stabbing, stinging, searing, racking, or tearing pain must be a

---

[1] *Bodily Sensations*, p. 119. [2] op. cit. p. 107.
[3] op. cit. p. 118. [4] op. cit. p. 119.

fairly *severe* pain. A pricking pain is milder.' This is quite plausible with words like 'searing' or 'racking'. We do not talk of searing sensations which are not pains, and a 'mild racking pain' seems a contradiction. This is because pains that 'sear' or 'rack' us are typically severe, in contrast with stinging sensations, which have a wider range of intensity, and pricking sensations which are characteristically milder. However, even though certain species of pain-sensations have a usual range of intensity, we should be careful before analysing them in terms of that intensity.

Armstrong has in fact confused three distinct questions. They do however lead into each other. He has failed to differentiate between the questions 'What sort of pain is it?', 'How intense is it?', and 'How much do you dislike it?' (or 'How much are you distressed by it?'). As we have seen, a stinging pain can have a wide range of intensity, and so to say that a pain is a 'stinging' one is to answer the first question, but not the second with any exactitude. Because a racking pain is typically severe, the word 'racking' appears to give an answer to both questions, and hence help to generate the confusion. There are, however, degrees of severity. It is ridiculous to assume that, having once docketed a pain as racking, we have fixed its intensity. A bad racking pain can always become an intolerable one, by an increase in its intensity. This leads to the connection between the second and third questions. Because a pain's increase in intensity is *almost* invariably a ground for our disliking it more, it is very easy to blur the distinction between the intensity of a sensation and our reaction to it. As a result, words like 'violent' and, to some extent, 'severe' carry with them the idea not only of an intense pain but of an intense pain we dislike. The intensity of pain is not the only ground we can have for disliking it. It is reasonable for someone to talk of preferring a searing pain to a racking pain, not because the one is less intense than the other, but because he finds the searing quality more bearable.

Armstrong's confusions are perpetrated in his attempt to do away with phenomenal entities and reduce bodily sensation to a species of perception. If his analysis of intensity in terms of disliking is to be rejected, as it must be, what account can be put in its place? What is it for a sensation to grow in intensity? It is a question that must be answered with regard to all sensations, and not just pains. Neutral sensations, such as throbs, which we may either like or dislike, still have intensity in the sense that some throbs are 'stronger' than others, and that each throb itself involves differences in intensity. Armstrong[1] says that 'throbbing pain rapidly waxes and wanes in intensity'. If that is so, presumably a throbbing sensation (or just a 'throb') does the same—and this once again prises apart intensity from dislike. It would be quite usual to say that one throb was more 'pronounced' than another, and this would mean more 'intense'. A more pronounced throb would be one which was more noticeable, and which made more demands on our attention. Cannot intensity be analysed in terms of the power of a sensation to make us notice it? In that case, the more intense the sensation was, the more difficult it would be for us to pay attention to other things.

The sensation's intensity cannot be analysed in terms of the attention we actually do pay it, as a very strong-willed person might be in intense pain and yet force himself to think of something else. The intensity would have to be understood in terms of the ease or difficulty with which he did this. At one end of the scale there would be extreme pain or 'agony' where a person's attention is swallowed up completely with the pain, and he finds extreme difficulty in thinking of anything unconnected with it. At the other end, a mild throb would be barely noticeable, and the more it grew in intensity, the more it would be liable to catch our attention.

It is possible to pay a great deal of attention to a mild pain, and this fact does not convert it into an intense one. Our reason, in that case, for saying that the pain was mild would be that we paid attention to it voluntarily, and that it would be possible to switch attention away from it without the sensation itself changing. An example would be a pain in the chest which a patient feared was a symptom of heart trouble. Worry about its significance might make him try to concentrate on the pain and to isolate its quality and location. The ease or difficulty with which he did this could be an indication of its intensity. If he had to shut his eyes to avoid being distracted from it we might assume that the pain was not very great. That it was not the pain itself but rather its significance that absorbed his attention

[1] op. cit. p. 119.

is shown by the fact that, if he came to believe an assurance by his doctor, that the pain was not a symptom of anything serious, he would give the pain as little attention as, say, a mild pain in his little finger. If he claimed that the intensity of the pain had not changed, although his beliefs about the pain had, we would have no reason to disbelieve him. We shall discuss this whole question again in Chapter VII with reference to the effects of prefrontal leucotomy.

The distinction between the pain itself and its significance is an important one, which might provide an explanation why, so far from being distressed at a pain, we sometimes appear to welcome one. An example would be someone who had a bad fall in a mountain accident, and was overjoyed at a bad pain in his leg, because it was a sign that his back was not broken, as he feared. This is not an example of someone actually *liking* pain. Other things being equal, he would certainly prefer to be without the pain than with it. Despite his joy, he may still have to brace himself to endure something which he does find unpleasant in itself. Here again, if his beliefs about the situation change, and he finds that the pain is not a good sign, his joy will disappear, and he will be left with dislike of, and even distress at, the pain. This suggests that there may be two distinct emotions, with different 'objects', at work. The joy is not joy at the pain itself, but at the situation. When the patient's view of the context of the pain changes, the 'object' of the joy is dissipated. Only the pain is left, and that is the 'object' not of the joy but of the distress and dislike which may have been overwhelmed by the man's great joy. The distress takes a simple 'object'—'the pain'— whilst the joy takes a propositional 'object'—'the fact that I am feeling pain'—and this has to be understood against a background of belief where 'feeling pain' is a good sign. This distinction between types of 'object' occurs even when we are only dealing with one emotion. I can take great joy in the fact that I am swimming (because, for example, I have been ill for a long time, and it is a sign that I can once more lead a normal life), while taking no joy at all in the swim itself (because the water is too cold).

It is obvious that an emotion such, as fear at the significance of the pain, will only serve to aggravate the patient's experience of pain—and an emotion like joy does serve to sugar the pill.

Psychologically both may be difficult to separate out from other elements in the pain experience, but this does not entail that it is logically impossible to do so. My fear may be centred on the pain, but I am not afraid of the pain itself, in the sense in which someone who knows he may not be able to endure it is afraid of pain. I am not concerned about the pain's possible effect on me. I am afraid that it is a sign of, say, heart trouble. It must be admitted that in some cases it is very difficult to distinguish between an 'object' of our emotion and its significance. Sometimes it may be a matter of viewing the 'object' in itself in one way, and its significance in another, with the consequent emotions fighting it out between them. Thus the man involved in the mountain accident might be overjoyed that he had not broken his back, and yet might still groan and wince at the pain which brought him his joy.

2. *Calmness and Emotion*

It was suggested earlier that the relationship between the intensity of a pain and dislike of it is a contingent one. If that is so it must be logically possible to have a violent dislike of a mild pain, and a mild dislike of an intense one. As we have seen, such cases may often turn out to be instances of some kind of emotional reaction to the significance of pain, rather than to the pain itself. It is very unlikely that one would have a violent dislike of a mild pain or vice versa, if only because the intensity of a pain is one of the main reasons we dislike it. The more intense it is, the less we are able to ignore it, and the more we dislike the quality of the sensations. Obviously our dislike can easily reach a pitch where it is natural to say that we are distressed. What of a patient who claimed of a pain that it was mildly unpleasant, but it didn't really bother him? He might say that he was calm and that his emotions were not involved. Would we have to point out that if the pain is mildly unpleasant, it follows that he does dislike it, and that an emotion is involved, even though it is a weak one?

There are in fact two related questions here. How far is calmness compatible with an emotion, and, secondly, is mere dislike an emotion anyway? First, it is possible for someone to be in an 'emotional state' (and it is interesting that this phrase definitely suggests a state of agitation) and still appear calm and collected. One can seethe with anger and still control its expression, though it would presumably require some effort. Similarly it is possible to be in severe pain, and still control any expression of one's agony, though if this was easy, it would suggest that one's suffering was not very great (and 'suffering' refers here as always to the emotional reaction to the sensation and not just to the sensation). Far more interesting are the cases where no great effort is needed to control the emotion or its expression. It was claimed at the beginning of the chapter that emotions are typically instances of excitement and disturbance. If this is so, can we apply the word 'emotion' to a situation where neither is present? If we do so too readily, the concept of emotion will be emptied of all meaning. Emotions, with their characteristic feelings, are distinguished from mere sensations by the fact that they have 'objects'. This, however, does not separate them from other mental states, such as thinking, which are obviously not emotions. The latter overwhelm us; we do not choose to adopt them, although we can put (or think) ourselves into a situation where it is likely that we will, for example, get angry. They have always been thought to be the enemy of reason rather than its adjunct. A man who acts in anger is acting as he feels he wants to because of something that has happened. He is not necessarily acting as he would think best if he reflected on the matter. His emotion may have clouded his judgement. Intense feelings and strong desires are typical of emotions; cool thought is not.

This is not to say that reason is not involved in emotion at all, or that emotions cannot be influenced by argument sometimes. Our beliefs about the situation and the way we view it are of immense importance. We cannot be in an emotional state if we are calm and collected, and an agitation of feeling (and of action) may serve to distinguish emotions from other attitudes. When, however, we have to decide what emotion we are feeling, our view of the situation is the deciding factor. An upsurge of feeling when I meet Mr. Jones may indicate that he sparks off some emotion in me, but I cannot say which one without considering what it is in my beliefs about him which arouse emotion. If I consider (rightly or wrongly) that he in some way embodies a threat to me, then I obviously view him with fear, whereas if I think that he has just done me an injury, then it is anger that I feel. There are many ways in which reason can dissipate my emotion. It may be shown me that I am mistaken about my facts. This man may not be Mr. Jones, or if it is, it may not be he who did me the injury. I may be wrong in my conception of what he did. On the other hand, my appraisal of the situation may be wrong, even if I do know all the facts. Someone could demonstrate that Jones' action was not detrimental to my interests, even though I had thought it was. If I altered my mind on any of these points my anger would be deprived of its grounds, and would usually vanish. It is interesting that, as an emotion which has a pain as its 'object' must be concerned with a genuine pain (I cannot wrongly believe that I am in pain), reason has very little scope for influencing the emotion.

Emotions always seem to arise as a result of something which I think affects either my interests or something I care about. If someone claimed to be angry at the rate the grass was growing and denied that this affected his interests in any way at all, but said that he was just angry about it, we would be nonplussed. If it meant that the speaker had to cut the grass before he wanted to we might understand, but if the sight of the grass getting longer day by day seemed to annoy him for no reason at all, what grounds would we have for admitting that he was angry? Even if he wanted it to stop growing and relaxed when winter came and it did, why should this be counted as anger rather than fear or any other emotion? Perhaps a psychiatrist might produce some explanation showing that the situation had a hidden significance, but then the patient could not be said to be angry at the grass growing, but rather at the significance which he conceived the situation as having.

Emotions often arise as a result of short-term selfish interests, and it is for this reason that they are rather untrustworthy guides to action. If I am indignant about something I think to be a personal slight, it might well be prudent from the long-term point of view not to give in to my emotion and the accompanying desires. On the other hand, some emotions might arise as a result of moral standards we care deeply about. Cruelty to a child or to an animal might arouse furious anger which might be completely justified. In this case I may strongly desire to put a stop to the cruelty, and as a result I may be said to think it is

a good thing to take action. Calm judgement will probably con-
cur with this. However, in the other case, I may want to
revenge myself for the slight inflicted on me and think it a good
thing to do so, but if the slight is put in context, and my own and
other people's long-term interests are brought into play, I may
realize that, in fact, it would be a very bad thing to do. Other
things being equal, if I want something, it is good for me to have
it, and if I do not want it, it is bad for me to have it. However
other things rarely are equal.

Professor Hampshire thinks[1] that what he calls the 'passions'
are constituted by 'the elements of pleasant or unpleasant affect,
and of reasoned or unreasoned thought'. He claims[2]: 'It is
important that fear, a representative passion, can be a calm
passion, in Hume's terminology, as well as a turbulent one, a
considered attitude as well as an uncontrollable perturbation.'
For him, the thought of something as dangerous is sufficient
for reference to 'fear'. He admits[3] that 'in the normal case' the
thought and the affect are combined, and the case in which the
thought alone is present must presumably be regarded as untypical and parasitic on more usual types of fear. Are we however justified in calling this kind of fear an 'emotion'? Not
every use of the word 'fear' can be regarded as such, precisely
because there is no element of agitation or disturbance. If
I reported that I took my umbrella because I was afraid of rain
I might certainly suggest that I thought rain was something
from which to be protected, but I could not be accused of getting in an emotional state about rain. My fears are not of the
kind which might grow until I was in a state of complete panic.
Hampshire himself[4] gives the example of 'being frightened of
German nationalism as a political force'. In this case one might
be in an emotional state about it and feel jittery whenever one
thought about it, but Hampshire envisages that it is a 'considered
attitude', mainly constituted by the belief 'that German
nationalism is in some way dangerous'. If, however, it is a
considered attitude, then it is not an emotion (or passion).
'Attitude' is a blanket word, which can cover all our thoughts
and feelings in a situation (usually as revealed in our actions).
Attitudes, so far from being contrasted with emotions, very often

---

[1] *Freedom of the Individual*, p. 97.
[2] op. cit. p. 85.
[3] op. cit. p. 97.
[4] op. cit. p. 84.

are emotions. My attitude to government policy could be one of furious anger. A considered attitude, however, is one which is not clouded by emotion, but has been carefully thought out, and deliberately adopted. It is not a spontaneous reaction to a situation as furious anger might well be. When, therefore, Hampshire suggests that 'calm passion' is equivalent to 'considered attitude' he is in fact saying that calm passions are not emotions, though he goes on assuming that a 'representative passion', such as fear, is *always* a passion (and he consistently uses 'passion' for such states as anger, fear, and terror, as an equivalent to 'emotion').

In fact Hampshire makes no distinction between a 'calm passion' and a 'mild' one. As we have seen, the first does not involve any disturbance or agitation, but is a rational and cool judgement. The second, however, does disturb us even if only a little, and our agitation could gradually become more pronounced. It is interesting to note that we do have a lot of simple names for states of non-agitation. 'Calmness', 'tranquillity', 'collectedness', 'coolness' are examples, and we might be tempted to call them emotions. However they are quite clearly used as the proper *opposites* of various emotional states, such as worry or anxiety. To talk of 'emotion recollected in tranquillity' is to contrast two distinct conditions.

3. *Dislike*

The first question—as to how far calmness is compatible with an emotion—has been dealt with. Calmness, in the sense in which a considered attitude is calm and involves no form of agitation, has no part in an emotional state. The second question, as to whether mere disliking is an emotion, must now be raised. There are some uses of 'like' and 'dislike' which are obviously not candidates as emotion. If someone claimed to dislike the foreign policy of Communist China, he need not be in any emotional state but could be delivering a considered judgement. He could be as calm as if he were saying that he disapproved of Chinese policy. His use of 'dislike' suggests that he considers that he—or something (such as his country) with which he identifies himself—is personally affected by it in some adverse way.

'Like' and 'dislike' can be used in a dispositional sense, and

here again they could not be termed emotions. They are not in
the same class in this respect as an emotion like anger, which
can be used in this way and still be termed 'emotion'. If I am
angry for a week, I need not be in an emotional state for every
minute. I need only be disposed to get into a rage, and do so
periodically. If, however, I dislike chocolate, I would not be
expected to shudder and generally become agitated while
periodically eating chocolate (although I might if I disliked it
a great deal and was forced to eat it). The mark of someone
with a dislike of chocolate is that he never puts himself in the
position of having to eat it in the first place. 'Disliking chocolate'
is in fact unlike 'being irritable' which is not an emotional state,
but a characteristic which means that its owner tends to get
into such a state easily in certain circumstances. Dislike of
chocolate involves a tendency to reject it.

This brings us to the basic point. If it is granted that 'disliking chocolate' is not an emotion in its dispositional sense,
could it be one in an episodic sense? If I dislike this bar of
chocolate, which I am eating now, am I in an emotional state?
There is no simple answer to this, partly because an almost
automatic reaction would be to spit it out, and not to get into
any state, however short-lived. If I went on eating it, without
being under any duress to do so, it would appear that I did not
dislike the chocolate. Unless I definitely would rather be without
something than with it and, *ceteris paribus*, take appropriate
steps to be rid of it, I cannot be said actually to dislike that
thing, although I could still 'not like' it. In fact a characteristic
feature of an episode of dislike must be a desire to be rid of the
'object' of dislike. The desire itself, however, could not be an
emotion. We do not experience emotion whenever we want
anything. My desire to buy a newspaper does not disturb or
agitate me, although it is possible that if I was continually
thwarted, my sense of frustration and of irritation would qualify
as emotional states.

The example of disliking pain, which is our main concern, is
free from the difficulties of 'disliking this piece of chocolate'.
We cannot choose to stop feeling pain (although we can of
course take steps which may rid us of it) and there is therefore
nothing paradoxical about continuing to feel it and disliking it.
It is the common lot of mankind. This very fact, however, might

make some refuse even to ask whether dislike of pain was an emotion. Pain, they might claim, is a reason for dislike and the two cannot be separated. Indeed we saw in the second chapter that a description of a sensation as painful is a completely adequate explanation for dislike of it (because, presumably, dislike of the peculiar quality of pain is so general). Vicious personal abuse almost invariably makes anyone angry although some may be better at controlling their emotion than others, and a person's awareness of a cruel insult inflicted on him would provide us with an adequate explanation of his anger. There is, however, still a clear logical distinction between knowing of an insult and getting angry about it, just as there is a distinction between feeling pain and disliking it. 'I become angry when vicously insulted' sounds just as odd as 'I dislike pain', and the reason is that the remarks state the obvious. It would be odd if the two situations did not arouse some reaction, as they so often do. We would expect to find some reason as to why they did not. The oddity is not a logical one however. The two remarks may be obvious, but they need not be analytically true.

This is a crucial point. It is very tempting to admit that emotions often have pain as their 'object' and still to maintain that dislike of the sensation should not be included on the emotional side at all. The distinctive quality of pain cannot, it is claimed, be separated from our dislike of it. If we do not dislike it, it cannot be pain, whatever a patient might say. Pain 'hurts', the argument goes. If it did not, it would not be pain. It is analytically true that we dislike what hurts. If we did not, what ground would we have for using the word? Therefore if we do not dislike a sensation it cannot hurt, and if it does not hurt it cannot be pain. Therefore logically we must dislike pain.

The trouble with this argument is that it demonstrates the logic of 'hurt' rather than 'pain'. It is quite true that the description 'it hurts' can only be applied to sensations with the quality of pain. Electric shocks are not usually said to hurt, even though they are unpleasant. Whether 'hurt' must logically connote dislike, or whether it does so only as a matter of fact because of the almost universal dislike of pain, is another matter. The fact that the word can also be used to suggest the infliction of distress or mental pain (as when I say that 'his words hurt me') indicates that it may have as intimate a connection with the emotional component of pain as with the presence of a sensation with pain-quality. This point however is somewhat counteracted by the possibility that this use is merely an analogical one, springing from the fact that pains 'hurt' (i.e. have 'pain-quality') and almost invariably arouse some sort of distress. As a result, any other 'object' of distress would be compared to pain and be said to 'hurt'. To say that his words hurt would in that case be to use the same kind of imagery as if I said, 'His words cut me to the quick'. There is probably no way of deciding which is the correct interpretation except by making an arbitrary ruling. One physiologist, Professor A. Forbes[1] is in no doubt. He talks of 'the threshold of what "hurts" (i.e. is unpleasant)'. He then attaches the word to the whole pain experience (sensation and emotion). However a philosopher, A. R. White,[2] obviously ties 'hurt' firmly to the quality of the sensation of pain. He feels able to write: 'The blow given in play hurts no less than that given in anger, yet we may enjoy it.' He sees no contradiction here and affirms that 'some people find pain satisfying for its own sake, they enjoy being hurt'.

If we decided that 'hurt' could only be applied when both the sensation with 'pain-quality' and an emotion such as distress were present, what would this show? It would entail that if we do not dislike or feel distressed at a sensation, we cannot use the word 'hurt', even if we recognize that the sensation has 'pain-quality'. It would entail that we could not use the word (and we do not) when we dislike a sensation which was not a pain. It would not mean that we must logically dislike pain, since to admit that not all pains hurt would no longer be self-contradictory. We would not be claiming that some pains do not have 'pain-quality', but rather that not all pains are disliked—as such dislike becomes one of the two necessary conditions for the use of the word.

A sensation with 'pain-quality', and our dislike of it, must each remain on opposite sides of the fence. However often they appear together, they *can* be separated logically. Is dislike, though, different from an emotion like distress, even if both are equally distinguishable from the sensation they have as 'object'? 'Distress' certainly suggests a great deal more disturbance and

---

[1] Quoted by H. K. Beecher, in *Measurement of Subjective Responses*, p. 158.
[2] *Attention*, p. 113.

agitation. Someone who was in pain, and in a distressed condition because of it, would have his attention almost swallowed up by the pain, and would certainly be far from calm. Someone, on the other hand, who merely disliked a pain but was not distressed by it, would be able to think of other things more easily, and would be able to behave in a much calmer way. It is important, however, that he would not be *completely* calm, as he would be if his dislike was a considered attitude. He would in some way be mildly agitated. Possibly his reaction might be only on the level of dislike, because the pain was short-lived, or moderate, or both. This dislike itself would not outlast its 'object' and would probably itself be mild, although the intensity of the dislike is not linked conceptually with the intensity of the pain. If the pain continued and at the same time slowly increased in intensity, it would be natural for the patient to get into a more obvious emotional state. If we wished to maintain that dislike was not an emotion (despite the fact that it is possible for emotions to be short-lived and mild) we would have to claim that at some point in the scale dislike became emotional. There would, however, be no obvious break when this happened. How could we tell when strong dislike became actual distress?

Someone might claim that even if it was not possible to make a clear line of demarcation, nevertheless we could do so notionally. Is not there an obvious difference between the distress of someone in intense and continous pain and the mere dislike of a twinge of pain by someone when he momentarily twisted his ankle? However all the criteria we have for the presence of emotion are present in both cases. The same kind of 'object' is present for both. The only real difference lies in the duration and degree of agitation. Is not there a similar comparison between a mild, and perhaps momentary, feeling of fear and a situation of continual and intense terror? Indeed the one can grow into the other in much the same way as dislike can grow into distress. Another example would be a state in which I am slightly peeved at someone. This could grow into one of furious rage. To feel mildly afraid or slightly peeved is not to be completely calm, or to have a considered attitude. They are mild agitations, like feeling dislike. It is interesting that the phrase 'to feel dislike' for someone or something is perfectly normal and idiomatic. Just as one can be said to have 'feelings of anger', so one can have 'feelings of dislike'. Even in this respect 'dislike' functions like the other emotions. Of course in the particular case of any emotion with pain as its 'object', as Brentano saw, any such feelings are unlikely to be noticeable, but would be 'fused into one' (psychologically not logically) with the pain. It was suggested earlier that emotions can only arise as a result of something which I think either affects my interests or something I care about, although it was pointed out that this need not be selfish. In other words, if I feel an emotion, I view its 'object' as being good or bad in some respect. To feel the emotion is to view the 'object' in that way. If, for example, I am afraid of something, I must logically view it as threatening me (or something connected with me) and as therefore bad, in this one respect at least. This means that it is very difficult to class surprise as an emotion, although in other ways it is very like one. It takes an 'object'. I cannot just be surprised. I must be surprised *at* something. Similarly a person who is surprised is not completely calm but is in some way 'agitated' or 'disturbed' (the latter word is perhaps the more appropriate for some emotions, such as 'object-directed' depression). Two features of an emotion are thus present. However, I do not necessarily view the 'object' of my surprise as good or bad for me. I am agitated because it was unexpected and not because I see it as beneficial or threatening in any way. It may be either of these, but in so far as I am surprised and not filled with joy or horror I do not view it as such. I am under no logical constraint to think that what is unexpected is good or bad in any respect. Similar considerations suggest that amusement is not an emotion. I can be amused at things which I realize do not affect me in the slightest and to which I am completely indifferent.

What of the emotions of dislike and distress, when they have pain as their 'object'? In what way do we view the pain when we dislike it or are distressed at it? Obviously dislike or distress involve the thought of something bad rather than something good. We wish to be rid of whatever we dislike. When we dislike pain, could it be that we are viewing the pain as a sign of damage? Undoubtedly pain does usually act as a warning-signal of bodily damage, particularly on the surface of the body, although it is often sadly disproportionate to the amount

5

of damage being done, and is sometimes absent when its presence would result in the saving of life. A toothache can be excruciating, whilst the early stages of cancer can be painless. The relevant question, however, is not whether pain is in fact linked with damage, but whether we view it as such when we react emotionally to it. If we discover that the 'object' of our fear is not in fact a threat, then we lose our fear. If we were told, when in pain, that although our pain was no doubt real enough we were in fact undergoing no physical damage, would our dislike or distress at the pain disappear? They surely would not. The connection of pain with damage might certainly exacerbate the whole experience in some cases, as the particular significance of a pain might at any time, but it would be a peripheral matter. What we dislike is the quality of the sensation of pain viewed in itself. Unless that is removed, our dislike is unlikely to be dissipated.

4. The 'Evil' of Pain

If we dislike a pain for its own sake, we think it bad, but this importation of the word 'bad' has its dangers. Just because pain is bad in this one respect—that we do not like it (or not usually) —it is not necessarily bad in every respect. We saw earlier that calm judgement may not necessarily agree that an action prompted by an emotion is in fact good in any respect other than in satisfying the limited desires connected with that emotion. In the same way, calm judgement may not follow the judgement implicit in an emotional reaction to pain. We may think it bad to have to endure pain in so far as we dislike it, and yet, when we put the pain in its context, we may very well conclude that it is positively good to endure it. For example, we may think it better to suffer pain in a dentist's chair and preserve our teeth, than to escape the pain and face the consequences of not having our teeth cared for. On a less trivial level, a martyr might think it better to endure pain then betray his faith, or a patriot suffering torture might prefer pain to the betrayal of his country. Any reference to the 'badness' of pain which is grounded merely on our dislike of it must contain a *ceteris paribus* clause, since other considerations might well be relevant. The omission of this clause enables philosophers to make unwarrantable logical jumps.

The basic trouble is that, when a philosopher has produced the thought 'the pain is bad' out of our dislike or distress at it, he tends to think he has proved more than he has. For example, D. M. Armstrong analyses the intensity of a pain in terms of our dislike of it, and our dislike in terms of how 'bad' it is and how much we want it to stop. He can therefore say[1] of a violent pain that 'we consider it a very bad thing, we have a very strong con-attitude to it', and of a mild pain that 'we consider it a somewhat bad thing, we have a weaker con-attitude to it'. We have already queried his attempted analysis of intensity in terms of strength of dislike. It by no means follows that we strongly dislike an intense pain, or only mildly dislike a moderate pain. Does the next stage in the argument hold good—namely that the degree of badness of the pain depends on the strength of our dislike? With the *ceteris paribus* included, this is unobjectionable, as we are not considering any ground for 'badness' other than dislike. Indeed in ordinary language we sometimes talk of a 'bad' pain and mean a pain we dislike a lot, or, as such pains are usually intense, a severe pain. However, to talk of a bad pain is not in any way to make a considered judgement or to evaluate it as I would be evaluating a man I called 'bad'. No argument could show me that the pain I was now feeling and disliking was not 'bad'. Yet Armstrong makes the jump from the viewing of pain as bad in one respect because of our dislike of it to a full-blooded evaluation of pain as 'an evil'. After recalling his analysis of the intensity of pain in terms of the strength of our dislike, he illustrates[2] by claiming: 'All things being equal, a pricking pain is a lesser evil than a stinging pain. And a prickle is a lesser evil still.' He presumably means that a pricking pain is less *bad* that a stinging pain, despite his sudden addition of 'all things being equal'. The words 'an evil' are normally reserved for fundamental obstacles to human interests and needs. Intense pain could be described as an evil because it tends to seize our attention, and make it impossible to satisfy our wants and achieve our ends as we would wish. If it were unnecessary, in the sense of not serving to warn us of injury to ourselves, it would presumably be an even greater evil. A mere pricking or a stinging pain, let alone a prickle, is hardly likely to be in this class.

[1] *Bodily Sensations*, p. 90.   [2] ibid., p. 119.

It would of course be possible to look at all the features of pain, and to conclude that out of them all it was man's dislike of it which made it so terrible for him, and that it was because of this that pain could be called 'an evil'. This would be very different from claiming that to dislike pain was actually to think of it as an evil. In that case, dislike of a pain would be the source of the proposition that it is an evil. In the former, it would merely be the reason for the judgement. Von Wright[1] takes this course and asks: 'Wherein does the evil of pain lie? To ask this is not to ask a triviality. Pain is evil, I would say, only to the extent that it is disliked or shunned or unwanted. It is a fact that pain is not always disliked.' It may well be true that dislike or distress at a pain is a necessary condition for its being judged an evil. However this may not be the only consideration. There are such points as the undoubted biological value of some pain. If pain did not distress us, or if we were congenitally insensitive to it, our failure to remove ourselves from pain-producing situations could injure us, perhaps fatally. It seems that our dislike of pain might even further our good sometimes.

Whether all pain, or only some, is evil, the crucial point is that such a judgement calls for the delicate comparison of different factors. It is not merely implicit in feeling distress, or dislike or any other emotion directed at pain. If it were, an argument which convinced me that the pain I was feeling was not an evil would be sufficient to dissipate my emotion.

[1] *Varieties of Goodness*, p. 57.

IV

'PAIN-REACTION'

1. *'Pain-Reaction'*

IT seems natural to talk of any emotion with pain as its 'object' as being a 'reaction' to pain, or if one wanted to be more specific an 'emotional reaction'. Unfortunately, the term 'pain-reaction' has been used in recent years to refer to anything from the central feeling of pain to remote consequences of the experience. As a result, considerable confusion has been engendered, and all too often a slide from one sense of the phrase to another has been made almost inperceptibly.

Emotional reactions to pain (and their associated desires), revealing a patient's attitude to his pain, are roughly what philosophers usually have in mind when they talk of 'reactions' in connection with pain. However, it must be admitted that they do not usually use the term 'emotion' themselves. For example, D. M. Armstrong[1] says:

Physical pain, in its typical manifestations at least, involves an immediate and interested desire that it should stop, and a loving concern for the painful place. It will be helpful to have a brief phrase to cover this whole complex of attitudes towards pain. Let us call it 'the pain-reaction'.

Armstrong explains that he means by 'loving-concern' that if our hand is hurting, we find that it absorbs our attention, and yet, though 'we are annoyed by the pain, we are not annoyed by our hand'. His reference to 'annoyance' at the pain suggests that the reaction is an emotional one.

Many physiologists would agree that emotions with pain as their 'object' should be included in the term 'pain-reaction', but they usually use the concept to cover much else besides. A modern textbook by Wolff and Wolf on the physiology of pain is a good example of this. They say[2]:

[1] *Bodily Sensations*, p. 94.　　　　　　　　　　[2] *Pain*, p. 21.

Included in the category of reaction to pain are not only disagreeable feelings, vocal and facial expressions of displeasure and alterations in sweating in the skin, but also, for example, the elevation of blood pressure. . . . Tachycardia and tapping of the feet are other reactions.

'Disagreeable feelings' do not presumably refer to the sensation of pain itself, but rather to an emotional reaction such as anguish. The other examples afford a peculiar mixture of bodily happenings which often accompany pain, but of which we are not usually aware, and straightforward pain-behaviour. Tachycardia, for example, is a completely different kind of pain-reaction from a groan or a grimace. Indeed such autonomic reactions, as distinct from pain behaviour, ought perhaps to be viewed as bodily responses to noxious stimuli, rather than as reactions of the individual to pain. It is significant that they occur in some (but not all) cases of congenital insensitivity to pain, where no pain is felt.[1] The tendency of some physiologists to talk of 'pain receptors' and 'pain pathways' may further the confusion. Although it may be convenient shorthand for receptors and nerve fibres, carrying impulses which can result in pain, after 'decoding' by the brain, this terminology is profoundly misleading. The impulses are not themselves pain, and to call them 'pain-impulses' can be dangerous. The natural result is to make the remark which Wolff and Wolf do[2]: 'Burning pain felt in the skin is transported like "cold pain" by fibres of small size which conduct more slowly.' Needless to say, pain is not 'transported' by fibres, although impulses are which may—and may not—result in pain. The idea that all nerve impulses which are the result of noxious stimulation are already 'pains' may blur the distinction between noxious stimulation and pain. It then becomes immaterial whether one talks of responses to noxious stimulation (which may occur when there is no feeling of pain) or of reactions to pain (which ought presumably to mean reactions to the *feeling* of pain).

What of such typical 'pain-behaviour' as what Wolff and Wolf call 'vocal and facial expressions of displeasure'? Such behaviour is an expression of an emotion (like distress) with

[1] See *Psychological Bulletin*, vol. 60 (1963): R. A. Sternbach on 'Congenital Insensitivity to Pain'.
[2] *Pain*, p. 7.

pain as its 'object', and as such it is merely the manifestation of one form of reaction to pain. It might appear that there was therefore a contingent relationship between it and pain, and here a difficulty arises. There is no standard cause for pain, although it is often associated with bodily damage. This means that the concept of pain cannot be taught merely by linking the sensation with a particular cause or type of cause. Instead it has to be taught through the sensation's connection with certain bodily behaviour. In addition, there is the difficulty that if the sensation of pain was not correlated in some way with publicly observable phenomena, there would be no guarantee that everyone meant the same thing by 'pain'. We must be wary, however, of emphasizing pain-behaviour too much at the expense of the 'quality of pain'. As we have seen, a willingness to give the name of 'pain' to many sensations, and yet to withhold it from such sensations as those produced by electric shocks (which might nevertheless be correlated with what was apparently pain-behaviour), suggests that a sense can be given to the concept of a 'pain-quality'. This brings us back, however, to the problem how this quality is to be linked with other features of the concept of pain by those who are being taught the concept.

2. *Pain-Behaviour*

A mother sees her child trip up, graze its knee badly and start crying. The features of the situation indicate to her quite clearly that he is in pain. She can then talk to him of the 'pain' he feels, and he thus begins to learn the concept. If he knocks himself badly and shows signs of distress, his mother will again refer to his 'pain', and he will himself come to recognize the distinctive sensations that occur in certain situations where he cries, winces or reacts in other characteristic ways. Because he has learnt the concept in such cases and shows he has understood it by referring to 'pain' when he does himself an injury and is distressed at it, we can accept his claims to feel a pain in situations when there is no obvious cause, or when he does not show by his behaviour that he dislikes the sensation in any way. We have no real check in such instances that he is using the word correctly, and so we have to rely for reassurance on this point on his correct use of the word in what we regard as paradigm cases of pain. It is this that enables us to accept claims of feeling pain, but not disliking it. What grounds could we have for rejecting them (once the concept of a pain-quality has been accepted) if we saw that on other occasions the word 'pain' was used quite normally by the very people who were now using it so strangely?

The importance of characteristic pain-behaviour in enabling the concept of pain to be taught is very real. A child who showed none of the usual 'pain-reactions' when he injured himself (in other words, none of the usual expressions of dislike or distress) would only be taught it with great difficulty on the basis of other people's behaviour, and even then would hardly understand the concept completely. If he invariably remained cheerful after a bad fall, it would be almost impossible to tell whether he felt pain, and did not mind it, or whether he did not feel pain at all. We shall discuss this more fully in connection with the problem of congenital insensitivity to pain. It is sufficient here to point out that unless there is a guide as to when someone is feeling pain, he can never be expected to 'catch on' to the distinctive quality of the sensations we call 'pain', because we could never be sure that we were using the word in a situation where he was in fact feeling pain. If, too, he showed no signs of distress, whenever he claimed to feel pain, we would be completely in the dark as to whether he and we meant the same thing by 'pain'.

Baier wishes to tie 'pain' completely to pain behaviour. According to him, if the behaviour, or at least an inclination to behave in that way, is absent, then what we feel is not a pain. He says of someone being taught the concept of pain:[1] 'Whatever he feels on the occasions when he naturally manifests pain he will learn to call "pain". And since he learns the word on the occasions when he feels something which he wants to stop, reduce in intensity, of whose return he is afraid etc. the very meaning of "a pain" will be "something which I dislike".' There is a certain amount of truth in this. Because pain is almost universally disliked, and because we depend on this fact to teach the concept, the word 'pain', as we have seen, can be used to refer to the whole pain experience of sensation and emotion. This, however, does not mean that there cannot be a secondary use of the

[1] *The Moral Point of View*, p. 275.

word, where it is used to refer to the sensation alone. Of course, this must be parasitic on the main use, as the sensation could not be called a sensation of 'pain' if the word had not been taught by means of characteristic pain behaviour. It is this which allows 'pain' to become a word in our common language. What we really mean if we talk of a pain which is not disliked is that the sensation has the same distinctive quality as those sensations which are the 'objects' of our dislike and distress (expressed in characteristic behaviour). Naturally we would be justified in expecting some kind of explanation as to why we normally dislike the sensation, but do not on this occasion (even if it is only a physiological one).

It must be concluded that, as our ability to teach the concept of pain is completely dependent on the behaviour which is the expression of our emotional reaction to pain, a purely contingent relationship between the sensation and our emotional reaction would be no basis at all for the existence of the concept. On the other hand, we have admitted the logical possibility of the sensation being recognized as pain and yet occurring without the reaction. This means that the connection cannot be a simple analytic one. It is a matter of logic, however, that if the concept of pain is to gain currency, the sensation and the behaviour must be correlated more often than not. Unless we can be certain that someone giving signs of distress in a situation normally productive of pain is more likely than not to be feeling pain, the word 'pain' can never come to be connected with the sensation. Just as the sensation can sometimes occur without the reaction, so can apparently typical pain-behaviour occur when there is no feeling of pain. Despite the appearances of the situation, the distress might have some 'object' other than a sensation of pain. This kind of case, however, logically must be abnormal. If it was quite usual, there would be no concept of pain. Not only could it not be taught, but, as we have indicated, there could be no guarantee that it was being applied correctly once it had been apparently learnt. The combination of pain and emotional reaction (and its manifestations) must provide the norm, and any deviations from it are logically secondary to it.

To disallow the possibility of any deviations from the norm within the concept of pain would be to provide ourselves with too blunt a philosophic instrument for dealing with abnormal cases, where there are indications that a patient might be feeling pain and yet be failing to react to it. Such cases do not fit our preconceived ideas about what it is to be in pain. They would not be 'paradigm cases' of pain. To deny, however, as Baier would, that they could logically be cases of pain is not to say anything more than that they are not normal instances.

3. Abnormal Cases

How abnormal a case can be and still be an instance of feeling pain is something that can only be decided by examining cases individually. In some instances, the various criteria we use for attributing pain may conflict to such an extent that we may be unable to make a definite decision. A case of hypnosis provides an example of this. Of all pain-reactions a patient's avowal of pain is obviously going to be of paramount importance to us in deciding whether he is feeling pain or not, provided that we have no reason to doubt his sincerity. It is tempting to say that a sincere avowal must be incorrigible, but what would a philosopher who argued for the incorrigibility of avowals make of a case where a patient simultaneously made two contradictory avowals, one that he was in pain and the other that he was not? He could not both be in pain and not be in pain at the same moment, and so it seems that one avowal must be wrong. The philosopher might feel his theory was safe, on the grounds that no one could make two opposite avowals at one and the same moment, and yet it looks very much as if that is what happens in the following case reported by E. A. Kaplan in an article on 'Hypnosis and Pain'.[1] The patient had been trained as a hypnotic subject.

A hypnotic analgesia for the left arm was suggested, and the subject was pricked in the left arm four times, with sufficient force to puncture the skin and subcutaneous tissues. After a minute or two, the subject asked the experimenter, 'When are you going to begin?,' apparently not having felt any pain. However from the moment that the pricking began, the subject's right hand had begun to write: 'Ouch, damn it, you're hurting me!'

Presumably the subject gave no other sign of pain in his behaviour, and this might incline us to believe what he said

[1] *Archives of General Psychiatry*, 2 (1960), 567–8.

rather than what he wrote. On the other hand, he had ample cause for feeling pain, and we would normally expect him to feel it in such circumstances, when he was not under hypnosis. Kaplan says: 'The subject's speaking voice seemed to be the organ of communication for that part of the personality (conscious?) which did not seem to perceive the pain, but the arm via automatic writing "spoke" for the portion of the personality which did perceive the pain.' This seems to suggest that the writing is in fact an 'avowal' on the part of an unconscious portion of the personality, but this is to say that the pain is 'unconscious' (or perhaps 'subconscious') and therefore unfelt, which involves us in a straight contradiction. We might conclude that the writing was not to be trusted and that the subject was not 'feeling pain'.

Another possibility might be that he did still feel pain, but that the hypnosis inhibited any inclination to state the fact in any normal way. Kaplan does admit the possibility in saying that hypnosis may merely 'facilitate denial by the conscious part of the personality'. In that case we would have to disregard what the subject actually said, as an example of a sincere avowal made erroneously. It is interesting, though, that our grounds for doing so would be another avowal of the same person, as it would be difficult to say that his writing was not an avowal even if it was made in a somewhat unconventional manner. Our philosopher who wishes to preserve the incorrigibility of avowals might suggest, in this case, that the spoken avowal (or perhaps we should say the avowal implied and entailed by the question 'When are you going to begin?') was not in fact sincere. However the subject's lack of any form of pain-behaviour might seem to support his sincerity. More important, the philosopher could have no grounds for claiming that he was insincere, other than the fact that he apparently made another avowal which contradicted it. It can be seen that all the philosopher has done is to reiterate his belief that sincere avowals are incorrigible. This avowal, his argument goes, has been shown to be incorrect. Therefore it must be insincere. This, however, is merely to beg the question as to whether someone can make contradictory avowals simultaneously, but in some sense be sincere in making both.[1]

[1] See p. 174 for a further discussion.

There are other spectacular types of cases of abnormal reactions to noxious stimuli where it is far from clear whether
the subject is feeling pain or not. Two of them, prefrontal
leucotomy and congenital insensitivity to pain, will be considered in subsequent chapters. Patients with psychiatric disorders sometimes present problems because of their lack of
reaction to stimuli which would be expected to produce pain
in normal people. Hall and Stride[1] report the results of experiments using an apparatus to measure pain by means of thermal
radiation. Waiving for the moment the difficulties inherent in
trying to 'measure' pain, we can examine the reactions to a
stimulus, intense enough to cause pain in normal subjects,
of patients classified as involutional-type depressives. The
authors say:

One patient in this category did not report pain even at the maxi-
mum intensity, but, on being asked to describe the nature of the
sensation, he said: 'Well, it was like a lighted cigarette-end being
held against my forehead.' This type of patient will frequently
describe a sensation as 'burning' or 'very hot' without, however,
making any admission that it was at all what they meant by pain.

Are these patients feeling pain (i.e. a sensation with 'pain-
quality') and not reacting emotionally to it, or are they not
feeling pain at all? They are obviously not 'in pain' in the
sense that they are having an experience of combined sensation
and emotion. The comparison by the patient between the sensation he was having and one he would have if a cigarette-
end was held against the forehead might suggest he was feeling
pain. Would it not be painful to have a lighted cigarette-end
pressed against one? The patient's refusal to use the word 'pain'
could be explained by a presumption that he was talking of
pain in the sense of sensation *and* emotion. The fact that he did
not mind the sensation would be for him sufficient reason for a
denial that he was in pain. This is possible, but very unlikely.
The patients obviously found nothing distinctive in the sensations besides the fact that they were 'burning' or 'hot' and as
the stimulus being used was thermal radiation, this is hardly
surprising. If their sensations were normal in every respect, in

the circumstances, apart from the fact that they did not have 'pain-quality', the patients' reports are precisely what we would expect. The thermal radiation gave them sensations of heat. The significance of the reference to the lighted cigarette-end would be merely that it was a comparison between two sensations of considerable heat. As the patients had presumably learnt the concept of pain in a normal way (their abnormal mental condition had not been life-long), their own refusal to call the sensations 'pain' must be decisive.

Hall and Stride dismiss the possibility that there is 'any difference in perceptual discrimination in these patients from that of other patients or of normal people'. They claim that the patients 'do, however, differ markedly in their evaluation of it as painful or not painful. This is demonstrated also by the fact that these patients report the stimulus as perceptibly warm, as early in the scale as most patients of similar age.' The reference to the stimulus is surely irrelevant here. It is not the stimulus, but the sensation caused by the stimulus, which is in question. The phrase 'evaluation of it as painful' is peculiar. As Hall and Stride are concerned to emphasize that these patients have the same feelings as others (or, to use their phrase, have the same 'perceptual discrimination') 'painful' is presumably not intended to refer to quality of a sensation, but is used as a synonym for 'distressing' or some such word. The claim is, therefore, that these patients are feeling the same kind of sensation as normal people but do not have any emotional reaction. The evidence Hall and Stride adduce supports our interpretation of their views. The fact that the patients feel warmth normally is intended to demonstrate that all their sensations must be normal. The authors' use of 'painful' to mean 'distressing' may be usual when what is described as painful is a situation, but in connection with sensations 'painful' is used to refer to a pain-quality—even if it may carry the idea that we are distressed by it. What they are doing is to define pain as 'a sensation which is disliked', and this has the result that they ignore their patients' inability to feel the distinctive quality of pain.

Cases of 'asymbolia for pain' provide interesting examples of an apparent divorce of the sensation of pain from any normal reaction to it. One case-history is reported by Hemphill and

Stengel[1] in a 'A Study on Pure Word-Deafness'. The patient had been admitted to hospital after a serious head injury, and the main feature of his condition seemed to be 'a lack of the ability to make an appropriate response to stimuli reaching the patient from the outer world'. This showed itself in a number of ways. He made no effort to get out of the way of a lorry behind him, despite the fact that, as he afterwards admitted, he had heard the horn and realized what it was. He tended to hear words and yet not understand them. We are told that 'the patient often complained that what he heard sounded like a foreign language, unknown to him'. This general characteristic also showed itself in his lack of reaction to pain. The authors report: 'When the patient was suddenly pricked, even very strongly, he failed to withdraw the part injured. There appeared to be a lack of the normal reaction of defence and flight from danger. He admitted that he could feel the painful stimulus for what it was.' Presumably by 'painful stimulus' is meant 'sensation of pain produced by the stimulus'. The authors continue by saying: 'During the examination the patient never failed to report on every single sensation and to describe correctly whether it was painful or whether it was innocuous.' It is unclear how they could ever hope to discover that the patient had failed to report on a sensation, unless he was trying to deceive them. If he sincerely denied feeling anything, how could Hemphill and Stengel contradict him, particularly as his lack of reaction would provide them with no evidence? It might be abnormal not to feel anything in the circumstances, but unless the authors are setting out with the conviction that he *must* feel something in certain circumstances whatever he may sincerely say, they cannot talk of 'failure to report sensations'. Much the same criticism can be applied to their reference to his describing *correctly* whether a sensation was painful or not. If he claimed his sensation was not one of pain, the authors could not tell him that it was—particularly as it is his ability to feel pain which is one of the points in question. All they can say is whether his claims to pain were normal or not. Presumably what they must be understood to mean, when they talk of his 'correct' reports as to whether he felt pain or not, is that his verbal response to stimulation of various kinds was quite

[1] *Journal of Neurology and Psychiatry*, 3 (N.S. 1940), 251–62.

normal. He said he was in pain when most people would say so, and denied that he was in pain in situations in which anyone would be expected to deny it. This is in itself important in reassuring us that he does know how to use the concept of pain. It is far easier for us to accept a claim to pain, when there is no reaction, if it occurs in a situation in which most people would feel pain. If someone said he felt pain, when, for instance, he was lightly touched by something and yet showed no signs of distress, we would have more reason to doubt whether he was using the word 'pain' in the same sense as we use it. Even in that case, however, it would be difficult to assert with conviction that he could not be feeling pain, if in other circumstances he used the word normally. If he said of someone writhing in agony after an accident that he was in pain, and at the same time claimed that he himself felt pain when anything brushed against him (although he said that he did not mind it and gave no sign of distress), it would be far from clear that he was ignorant of the concept in any way. Perhaps he might be the victim of some strange physiological disorder.

To return to the case of asymbolia for pain, it is significant that the patient soon realized that his lack of reaction to pain was interesting the examiners, and he felt a need to explain it. It looks as if he understood the concept of pain well enough to realize that failure to react to pain was abnormal. In these circumstances it is all the more important that, despite his knowledge that he was not reacting to pain, and despite an understanding that this was odd, he still insisted that it was 'pain' which he was feeling. Hemphill and Stengel report: 'He tried to explain his reactions by such expressions as: "I am not a man who cannot stand pain" or "I am used to that, because I have worked on the road" or "labourers are always hurting themselves: we don't take any notice of it". On the other hand his wife assured us that he had always been susceptible to pain and had reacted violently whenever his children pricked or pinched him in play.'

This seems to be a clear case of someone who had sensations, which he recognized as being of pain, and yet who did not react emotionally to them in any way. Any suggestion that he must have misused the word 'pain' is rebutted by his obvious worry that he was not reacting normally. He knew that it was usual for people in pain to show signs of distress, and that some explanation for his lack of 'pain-reaction' was called for. One solution would have been that what he was feeling ought not to be called 'pain', and the fact that he did not take this easy course must make us ready to accept his claim. His sensations must have had a very distinctive quality, which he thought could only be classified adequately by calling them 'pain'. Obviously it was the quality which he usually associated with typical pain-reactions.

Another explanation which might be put forward to pre-serve the connection even in this case between pain and dislike could be that the abnormality did not lie in his lack of dislike of a sensation of pain. Instead it might be suggested that he did dislike the sensations (and this might be the reason he called them 'pain'). The abnormality might rather consist in his inability to react in a normal way to a sensation he disliked, and to which therefore he had a felt inclination to react. A parallel could be drawn between this and his lack of reaction to a lorry horn which he nevertheless realized was meant to warn him (although it is not clear how far he realized he ought to take any action as a result). However his explanations as to why he did not react do not imply that he had any inclination to do so. What he is obviously explaining by such phrases as 'I am not a man who cannot stand pain' is his lack of desire to react to the pain. He is not giving a reason as to why his desires mysteriously do not get transformed into action. To say of pain that labourers 'don't take any notice of it' is to say that they do not mind it, that it does not bother them. It is not to say that they are distressed by it, but stoically do not let their feelings show. Similarly his claim to be 'used to' pain suggests that he is not disturbed by it in the slightest.

There is a complete difference between this case and another, which is reported by Rubins and Friedman.[1] They tell of a woman who 'when severely pricked to the point of drawing blood would say "ouch" and occasionally grimace, but never withdrew her limbs or turned her head away'. This looks far more like a case where the patient is somehow inhibited from expressing in her behaviour a very real dislike of the pain. Her

[1] *Archives of Neurology and Psychiatry*, 60 (1948), 554-73.

exclamation and grimace are at odds with her lack of withdrawal of her limbs. On the other hand, it appears likely that
her dislike of the pain was considerably less than normal. The
fact that it took severe pricking to make her show any sign of
pain would indicate this, although it is possible to maintain
that this too was a part of her general inability to express her
reaction to pain. Rubins and Friedman also report other cases,
and they say: 'The degree of response to the stimulus varied
from complete denial of the pain to verbal exclamation after
stimulation and finally to some partial movement of escape.
Two patients stated repeatedly that the pinprick did not hurt
even after prolonged application and to the point of drawing
blood.' It is unclear whether a denial that something 'hurts'
amounts to a denial of pain. Is the patient saying that what he
is feeling is not a sensation with 'pain-quality', or is he just
saying that he does not mind the sensation? Rubins and
Friedman do not consider the possible ambiguity of the word
'hurt', as they do not see the distinction between being able to
feel a pinprick and being able to feel a sensation with 'pain-
quality'. If a patient is not numb they assume that he can feel
pain, and all interest must then centre on the patient's ability,
or lack of it, to react normally to pain. They make this quite
explicit when they say of one case: 'Pain sensation as evaluated
by our routine criteria—namely ability to distinguish between
sharp and dull on application of a pointed object or to perceive
sharpness with the same intensity—was normal'. These criteria, however, have nothing to do with feeling pain. We have
seen that certain types of mental patients can be subjected to
this kind of stimulus, and still deny pain (and the same holds
true of those who are congenitally insensitive to pain). Such
cases may be very odd, but surely they are intelligible. It is in
no way self-contradictory to report sensations of sharpness
normally, and yet to deny pain. Just because such sensations
may normally possess the quality of pain, it does not follow that
they must always. Rubins and Friedman can be accused of
paying too much attention to the nature of the stimulus, and
not enough to the nature of the sensation, as described by the
patient. Because a stimulus, such as severe pin-prick, is normally painful, they assume that all that is required for the
occurrence of pain is that the patient perceive the stimulus.

6

They forget that it is possible for the sensations produced by the same stimulus to vary.

Because of this, it is impossible to decide whether the cases fall into the same category as that reported by Hemphill and Stengel. Are the patients feeling a sensation with the distinctive quality of pain, or, like the psychiatric patients, are they really perceiving the stimulus, but not feeling pain?

4. *Conceptual Confusions*

We have been examining various examples of abnormal reactions to normally painful stimuli, and have been attempting to decide how far they are instances of abnormal reactions (or a lack of reaction) to a sensation of pain. The occurrence of a stimulus which normally produces pain is not a sufficient condition for feeling pain (indeed it is not a sufficient condition for feeling anything). Yet it is all too easy for physiologists to jump from a 'normally painful stimulus' to 'pain', or from a 'reaction to the stimulus' to a 'reaction to pain'. This sometimes has bizarre results. Pain, of course, can be described as a reaction to a stimulus. For example, Sauerbruch and Wenke[1] claim: 'Just as pain is a reaction to local stimuli so anxiety is a reaction to real or imagined danger.' This comparison itself foreshadows a confusion often perpetrated between different types of reaction. The reaction of pain to a stimulus is not an emotional reaction, while anxiety is. It involves no view of the stimulus, as anxiety must involve a view of its 'object'. The proper comparison would have been between distress at pain and anxiety at real or imagined danger. As it is, it is almost suggested that the stimulus is an 'object' of pain, and this is obviously ridiculous, not least because one does not have to know the cause of the pain to feel it. 'Pain-reaction' in fact is an umbrella concept which shelters two distinct ideas. It is possible to use it to mean a reaction *of* pain to some stimulus, and it can also mean an emotional reaction *to* the experience of pain. If these are confused, one can easily come to the surprising conclusion that one of the reactions *to* pain *is* pain.

This kind of shift from stimulus to sensation, and from the reaction to one to the reaction to the other, is clearly seen in the work of Dr. H. K. Beecher, who has, more than any other

---

[1] *Pain—its Meaning and Significance* (trans. E. Fitzgerald), p. 68.

physiologist, emphasized the importance of the 'reaction component' in pain. Our text will be his own summary of his views[1] in the Symposium on *The Assessment of Pain in Man and Animals.*[2] Here we read[3] that 'processing of a stimulus has occurred by the time a noxious stimulus erupts—or is prevented from erupting—into consciousness.' However what we feel is not a stimulus but a sensation caused by a stimulus. Beecher is evidently uneasy about his use of 'stimulus' in this way, and switches to talking of sensations. He says:

One can generalise with great likelihood of truth by saying no psychological sensations are pure; they are all modified by processing. Better then to speak of perceptions than sensations. These include processing, reaction, based among other things, on the personality, on past experience, on present significance, on meaning to the conditioned individual.

Beecher divides[4] 'pain' into two components—the 'original sensation' and the 'reaction to the original sensation'. If, however, 'reaction' is a synonym for processing, it is difficult to see what sense can be given to the words 'original sensation'. Presumably the nerve-impulses set in train by some stimulus are what Beecher has in mind, but to call these 'sensations' is as misleading as to talk of 'pain pathways'. It is self-contradictory to talk of 'unfelt sensations' and 'unfelt pains', and yet we would be forced to if we followed Beecher in equating sensations with nerve-impulses. These have to be 'decoded' by the brain before they become pains, and to call the process of 'decoding' and interpretation 'reaction to pain' is misleading, even if factors other than the nerve impulses are involved. We can see that the process by which we feel pain, as a reaction to a stimulus, has already been dubbed 'a reaction to pain'.

Beecher makes his confusion quite explicit by proceeding to use the words 'stimulus' and 'sensation' as synonyms. He talks[5] of the 'working concept of an original sensation, an original stimulus, and the psychological reaction to it'. Even his use of the word 'stimulus' is ambiguous. He claims that, when talking of the psychological reaction components, he does not mean a physical reaction to a stimulus, as the swift removal of a

[1] To be found in extended form in his *Measurement of Subjective Responses.*
[2] Ed. Keele and Smith, pp. 159–69.   [3] op. cit. p. 162.
[4] op. cit. p. 161.   [5] op. cit. p. 164.

burned finger from a flame'. Presumably, he regards the flame as a typical example of a stimulus, liable to produce pain. Yet the flame is surely not the same thing as a 'sensation', even if one allows Beecher's misuse of 'sensation' for a moment. The kind of 'stimulus' which he envisages as being synonymous with his use of 'sensation' must, as we have suggested, consist of nerve impulses. Just as these are not a sensation, so a flame is not a nerve impulse, although it would usually cause one. He has run together three separable items in a causal chain (stimulus, nerve impulses, and sensation).

With these confusions as a basis, Beecher goes on to include in the apparently unambiguous concept of pain-reaction both reactions *of* pain to stimuli, and emotional reactions *to* pain. In a summary of the evidence for the existence of the reaction component he remarks[1]: 'It is common observation that emotion can block pain.' He then goes on to say: 'Differentiation between pain and comfort, whether by lobotomy or by drugs, supports the concept under discussion.' However, these two statements are each evidence for a different concept. The first shows that in circumstances when one feels strong emotion (or, as Beecher adds elsewhere, when one is distracted) one might not feel any pain at all. He quotes his experience at Anzio[2] in the Second World War, where only 'one-quarter of the severely wounded men . . . had enough pain to want anything done about it—and this affirmation was made in response to a direct question which was of course suggestive.' He puts this down to the euphoria of many of the men at being released from an intolerable situation. If this is genuinely a case of emotion blocking pain (as opposed to one of just not minding the pain they did feel because it meant the war was over for them) it is a matter of physiology. It shows that pain does not necessarily dominate the nervous system. 'Central control of peripheral perception' (to quote Beecher again[3]) is no doubt worth emphasizing, and the active part being played by the brain in dealing with nerve-impulses is being recognized more and more. This has, however, nothing to do with the influence of lobotomy (or leucotomy as it is now generally called) and

---

[1] Ed. Keele and Smith, p. 165.
[2] op. cit. p. 163, and see also H. K. Beecher, *Annals of Surgery*, 123 (1946), 96–105.   [3] op. cit. p. 162.

drugs. These, as we shall see in subsequent chapters, are held to affect the emotional reaction to pain, and do not affect what sensation we feel.

Beecher claims[1]: 'The reaction to a stimulus is influenced by the subject's concept of the sensation, by its significance, its importance, meaning, or degree of seriousness.' Once again, we have the explicit shift from a 'stimulus' to a 'sensation', but this time Beecher really does mean 'sensation' in its proper use, as is shown by the example he gives. He goes on to say: 'One pain, as beneath the sternum, if it connotes sudden death can be wholly unsettling: a pain of the same intensity and duration in a finger can easily be disregarded.' He is talking here of comparative attitudes to two similar *pains*, and not to two similar stimuli. It may well be that anxiety and fear about the significance of a pain should be included in the concept of 'pain-reaction', but it should be noticed that this is not the same type of emotional reaction as distress at the pain itself (because of its quality or intensity). In the third chapter we distinguished between a pain and its significance, and the distinction must be applied to this example. Beecher postulates that the two pains are similar in all respects except location (and hence significance), and that the pain in the finger can 'easily be disregarded'. This must mean that it is not very intense. The other pain does seem to be an 'object' of powerful emotion, and here our distinction must be applied. If it is *ex hypothesi* similar to the other pain, it can be concluded that in itself it is not the 'object' of great distress. Its significance, however, is clearly the 'object' of considerable anxiety. If our beliefs about this were changed, we would be as little bothered about this pain as we would be at the pain in our little finger. Despite the reduction of our anxiety, the pain and our dislike of it need not be affected in the slightest, although the total psychological experience of pain and the various forms of emotional reaction to it and its significance will change markedly.

We have two general categories of emotional reaction to pain, distress at the pain itself, and anxiety at its significance. The distinction is relevant to Beecher's discovery[2] that narcotic drugs have a far more dependable effect on 'pain of pathological origin' than 'pain of experimental origin' (i.e. pain

[1] Ed. Keele and Smith, p. 164.   [2] op. cit. p. 165.

produced artificially in a laboratory for experimental purposes).
He says:

Experimental methods unquestionably produce real pain (but not
pain dependably relieved by the usual dose of narcotics) and since
this probably more nearly represents 'original sensation' (less
significant, less processing) than is true with pathological pain, one
is left with the working hypothesis that certain drugs, analgesics,
for example, primarily act on the reaction component.

In bringing up again his peculiar concept of an 'original
sensation' Beecher becomes involved in another confusion,
although one that is closely connected with his previous ones.
To say of a sensation that it has been 'processed' less than
another is not to say that it is less significant, and vice versa.
The two descriptions refer to different stages in the feeling of
pain. The first is a physiological point, the second is not. It is
easy enough to see how this particular error arose. If Beecher
fails to differentiate between the physiological 'processing' of
nerve impulses, and the emotional reaction to a pain, and if he
does not distinguish between the two types of emotional reaction (distress and anxiety), it becomes logical for him to
assume that the physiological processing and anxiety at the
significance of a pain are identical.

His failure to realize that distress at a pain is not at all the
same emotion as anxiety (or fear) at its significance, because
their 'objects' are quite distinct, does leave a question which is
not asked. Do narcotics relieve our anxiety, do they lessen our
distress, or do they do both? This ought to be an important
question for Beecher. He believes that certain drugs 'primarily
act on the reaction component' (although it has been a matter
of dispute amongst pharmacologists whether they do raise the
'threshold' of the sensation of pain). It thus is relevant to ask
which part of the reaction component is influenced. His assertion that pain of experimental origin is 'less significant' may
well be true. It could hardly be viewed as a sign of disease by
the person who felt it, and he would be well aware that it
would pass when the experiment is over. There would hardly
be any grounds for anxiety or fear of the future, although presumably dislike of the sensation itself would be present. Are
narcotics successful, therefore, with pathological pain because
they relieve anxiety, and less successful with experimental pain

because there is little anxiety there in the first place? This seems to be what Beecher is implying, and it is the absence of anxiety which leads him to talk of the pain which is produced by experimental methods as being more nearly 'original sensation' We are entitled, therefore, to ask what, according to him, are the effects of drugs on distress at the sensation itself. Can we, as a result of the influence of a drug, feel a pain and not dislike it, or is it just our anxiety about its context which is relieved? Because Beecher wrongly regards his concept of 'reaction component' as single and indivisible, he cannot ask this question.

V

'THE SAME SENSATION'

1. *The Analogy between Pains and Visual Experiences*

WE have seen that a sensation can sometimes be separated
from our normal reaction to it. A new question now presents
itself. If our reaction to a sensation changes, what grounds
have we for insisting that we do still feel 'the same sensation'?
This is particularly difficult in the case of pain, where the sensation tends to be associated with a particular type of reaction,
and where, indeed, the name for the sensation is taught by
means of the reaction. It becomes all too easy to say dogmatically that if the sensation is not disliked it cannot be pain. If
we do this, we are still faced with insistent claims that it is
'the same sensation'.

Some philosophers are tough-minded about questions concerning the sameness of sensations. Kenny (taking an unduly
simple view of masochism) asks[1]:

Does whipping cause the masochist a different sensation from the
ordinary man, or does it cause him the same sensation, which he,
unlike the rest of us, happens to like? To this question, one answer is
as good as the other; which shows that there is no possibility of
setting up criteria for the sameness of sensations independently of
what causes them and what people do about them.

According to Kenny we are tempted to call the sensation
'pain' because it was caused by whipping, a normal cause of
pain, but we are forced to hesitate because of the absence of a
normal 'pain-reaction'. Our two criteria point in opposite
directions. How therefore can we make a decision at all? Presumably Kenny would take the same line with any case where
our sensation of pain appeared to be separated from a normal
reaction. The same kind of problem arises with other types of
sensation. It is a matter of common experience that if one

[1] *Action, Emotion and Will*, p. 143.

drinks a cup of tea thinking it is coffee it has a horrible taste. Immediately one realizes that it is tea, it is possible to enjoy it. Does the taste change when we find out what we are drinking, or does it remain the same, while our attitude to it changes? At one moment we dislike the sensation in our mouth, but when we know what we are drinking, we like it. Just as with the cases of 'pain', the cause of the sensation would incline us to answer one way, while our reaction to it would suggest the opposite. We would expect the same cup of tea to keep the same taste from one moment to the next. On the other hand, it might be thought usual to react in the same way to the same sensation, and a change in reaction would often be a good indication that the sensation has changed. This latter point cannot be pressed too far. We talk of 'acquiring a taste for something' and this just means coming to like a taste which we previously did not care for. It is a reasonable assumption that the taste has not changed in such instances. It is perfectly intelligible to suggest that, although a child does not like the bitter taste of coffee, he will grow to like it, even though it will still taste as bitter. This is exactly what we might expect, if it is possible to separate sensations logically from our reactions to them. Unless a sensation is linked indissolubly with one kind of reaction, it will be logically possible to like or dislike it, *per se*, without it changing in any way. Indeed it is obviously ludicrous to claim that we must, for example, like the normal taste of tomatoes. It would follow that if we did not like the taste when we ate some, the taste could not be the usual one. The difference in reaction to the taste would entail that the taste itself was different. This might on occasion be so, but we are under no logical compulsion to assume that tomatoes must have an abnormal taste for someone who dislikes them. He can surely dislike them just *because of* the taste which they normally have.

Wittgenstein wrestled with an analogous problem in the second part of the *Philosophical Investigations*.[1] He was particularly concerned then with the problem of ambiguous drawings, which could be interpreted in more than one way, such as the drawing of the 'duck-rabbit' which can be seen as a rabbit's head or as a duck's. Do we see the same thing, when we

[1] II. xi, pp. 193 ff.

interpret the drawing first as a rabbit, and then as a duck, or does our 'visual experience' itself change? Wittgenstein asks:[1] 'Do I really see something different each time, or do I only interpret what I see in a different way? I am inclined to say the former. But why?' A perplexing feature of the duck-rabbit is that, if asked to draw what they saw, someone who saw the figure as a rabbit and someone who saw it as a duck could well produce exactly the same drawing. Each of them could nevertheless still be unaware of the alternative interpretation. This gives us a reason for saying that they saw the same thing. On the other hand, Wittgenstein says[2]: 'I see two pictures with the duck-rabbit surrounded by rabbits in one, by ducks in the other. I do not notice that they are the same. Does it *follow* from this that I *see* something different in the two cases?' He refuses to admit that it does follow, but merely says: 'It gives us a reason for using this expression here.' We thus have reasons both for saying that we do see the same thing and that we do not. Wittgenstein presses the question as to what is different, and asks whether his 'impression' or his 'point of view' has changed. To this he merely retorts: 'Can I say?' As with pains and tastes, we have conflicting criteria, and Wittgenstein refuses to make a decision. Instead he suggests[3] that the criterion of the visual experience is 'the representation of what is seen', and goes on to claim: 'The concept of a representation of what is seen, like that of a copy, is very elastic, and so together with it is the concept of what is seen.' We can hope for no precise answers as to whether what we see is the same or not, when we interpret the same drawing in different ways.

Wittgenstein claims[4]: 'Here we are in enormous danger of wanting to make fine distinctions. . . . What we have rather to do is to *accept* the everyday language-game.' We cannot answer questions about whether we are seeing something different when we see a duck, from when we see a rabbit. We may persist in wanting to know whether we do really have a different impression, and Wittgenstein says[5]: 'How can I find out? I *describe* what I am seeing differently.' That is all that can be said. If we still have reasons for saying that we are seeing the

[1] II. xi, p. 212.   [2] op. cit. p. 195.
[3] op. cit. p. 198.   [4] op. cit. p. 200.
[5] op. cit. p. 202.

same thing (because, for example, our drawings of the duck and the rabbit were identical), we can make no final decision.

It has been found in psychological experiments that the shape of a familiar object will lead observers to expect that the shape possesses the normal colour of that object. If subjects are shown the shape of a leaf and the shape of a donkey, cut out of the same material, and are asked to match the exact shade from a colour wheel, they will tend to indicate a greener shade for the leaf, and a greyer one for the donkey. We are naturally led to ask whether their expectations lead them to see slightly different colours from those which are in fact in front of them. Are their 'visual impressions' different from when they look at a sample of the same colour in no particular shape? Wittgenstein might claim that we had no way of deciding, and that we should not be tempted to make such fine distinctions. We have a reason for saying that the shape affects the way we see the colour, and that is as far as we can go.

It can be seen that Kenny's approach to the masochist's 'pain' is very similar to Wittgenstein's approach to the duck-rabbit. The fact that the masochist's sensation was produced by whipping gives us a reason for calling it 'pain'. The fact that he shows no 'pain-behaviour' gives us a reason for not calling it that. We must accept the everyday language-game, and not try to make fine distinctions. We are faced with conflicting criteria, and that is that. This has a certain degree of plausibility with the duck-rabbit and similar cases. It also seems a possible way of dealing with the bewildering case of the tea which we think is coffee. Should we say that at one moment we found the taste horrible, and the next we found it pleasant, or should we rather claim that the taste of the drink changed from being a horrible one to being a pleasant one? The first version suggests that the taste in our mouth remained the same while our attitude changed, and the second indicates that the taste itself changed. There seems no way of telling which is right. If someone insisted that the taste did remain the same, although they no longer disliked it now that they realized what they were drinking, we would have our puzzle solved. Their assertion would give a clear sense to any talk of the sameness of the sensation. Our difficulties arise if they are unwilling to do this, and are reluctant themselves to make a decision. On either

interpretation at least one of the elements in their experience
has changed, and they may not differentiate between them.
They like tasting liquid which they previously did not like, and
that is all they know. In this they are in a similar condition to
viewers of the drawing of the duck-rabbit. It looks different
when they see it as a rabbit from when they see it as a duck,
but they cannot say whether this is because of a difference in
what they see, or in the way they interpret it. We are not in the
position of wondering whether what they say can be right, but
rather of trying to decide for them what they ought to say.

There are cases of illusion where a person's expectations or
beliefs seem quite clearly to govern what they do see, and where
such a person is quite definite in telling us. Indeed it is this
certainty, coupled with an assurance on our part that he does
have a good grasp of, say, colour concepts, that gives a sense to
the whole concept of illusion. If we thought that someone's
claim to see a colour which was not in fact in front of him was
an example of a general inability to distinguish some colours,
we could just dismiss what he said as a mistake. If, however, he
had previously named colours accurately, we can accept that
he is reporting some abnormal experience. An example is
given by E. H. Gombrich in *Art and Illusion*. He quotes the
following[1]:

I was looking out of the window, watching for the street car, and I
saw through the shrubs by the fence the brilliant red slats of the
familiar truck; just patches of red, brilliant scarlet. As I looked, it
occurred to me that what I was really seeing were dead leaves on a
tree; instantly the scarlet changed to a dull chocolate brown. I went
out to see what the colour really was, and found it to be a distinctly
reddish brown.

It would seem strained to suggest that the writer saw the
reddish brown quite normally and interpreted it as red and
then brown. Until he went out and looked at the colour from
close quarters, how could he be said to be seeing reddish brown
(except in the trivial sense that what he saw was in fact reddish
brown)? He obviously had a full command of colour concepts,
so much so that he realized the oddness of his experience. As a
consequence, his claims to see red and then brown must be

[1] p. 189 (quoted from an article by G. K. Adams).

respected. There is no question here of a conflict of criteria. What we are faced with is an abnormality, the cause of which must be explained by science. We can define what a person thinks he sees as the 'object' of his sight (although we must continue to be wary of the misleading implications of the term). In this case the red and the brown which the writer thought he saw were the 'objects' of his sight, while he was in fact looking at reddish brown. Once we recognize his grasp of colour concepts, a man's own claims as to the colours he is seeing will alone establish whether the 'object' of his vision is identical with the material object. What he says that he sees is the only criterion we have with which to judge what the content of his visual experience may be. If he says that the colour that he now sees is the same colour as, say, a London Transport bus, then whether the colour of the thing in front of him is the same or not, we must accept this is a true description of his present experience. We must do the same if he claims that the colour he sees is the colour of chocolate.

This position is analogous to the one which can be adopted over the abnormal claims of someone to feel pain, even though he liked the sensation, or, at any rate, did not dislike it. Provided that he has demonstrated an adequate knowledge of the use of the word 'pain', his application of it in an abnormal situation need not be a mistake. It is important to stress that this does differ from the colour case in one respect. We would not say he was suffering an illusion. That concept would be completely inappropriate here. There are no such things as illusory pains, since there is no way of distinguishing an illusory pain from a real pain. We cannot appeal to the experience of others to help us decide whether we are undergoing an illusion, as we can with colours. We can be told that what we see as red is in fact reddish brown, because others, in normal conditions, claim to see it as reddish brown. The red is not 'really there'. We are all looking at 'the same colour' and the judgement of a person in normal conditions with normal sight sets the standard. If I claim to see scarlet, I am making a mistake about what the colour in fact is, although I am not making a mistake about my visual experience. I do see it as scarlet, but it is not scarlet. My pain is thus in the same kind of category as that of a visual experience, and not that of a colour. I will not withdraw my

description of my visual experience when I agree that I was
not seeing scarlet, in the sense in which the scarlet would be
there for myself or other people to see in normal conditions
(and without any special belief that I am looking at, for instance, a red bus). Similarly, I will not withdraw my description of my pain, despite my discovery of any abnormality. I
may think that the pain is in a limb which has in fact been
amputated. If I find out that I no longer have the limb, I will
not withdraw my claim to feel pain. Similarly if I realize that
the cause of my pain is not a usual cause of pain for anyone,
and that others in similar circumstances are not talking of
pain, I will not necessarily withdraw my claim. It is possible
that I am abnormal. Failure to conform is not itself fatal to my
claims to pain. I am not expected to fall back on saying that I
thought I felt pain, as I would say that I *thought* I was seeing
scarlet, if no one else agreed with me about the colour, or if I
myself from a different point of view, or without any of my
previous preconceptions, realized I had been wrong about
what the colour really was. The writer we quoted who was
looking out of the window was in this latter position. My
thought that I was feeling pain would not be a peculiar kind
of pain experience which can be distinguished from actually
feeling pain. If I think I am feeling pain, then I am feeling pain.

It would appear that our criteria for talking of the 'same
visual experience' and the 'same pain' are very similar. Once
the person is seen to understand the relevant concepts, if he
says without any intent to deceive that he is feeling the same
pain, then he is feeling the same pain. In the same way, if
he says that he has the same visual experience as he gets if he
looks at a London Transport bus or a British pillar-box, then
we can understand that he is seeing red, whether there is something red in front of him or not. The basic puzzle about the
duck-rabbit and the tea which we think is coffee is that people
seeing the drawing and tasting the drink can themselves make
no clear decision about their experiences, and make no definite
claim about whether they are having the same visual experience
with different interpretations of it, or the same taste with different attitudes to it. The other example quoted, of a material,
the colour of which we see differently according to its shape,
is an easier one to deal with. People looking at the different

shapes would claim to see slightly different colours, as can be seen by their choice of different shades from the colour wheel.

2. The Classification of Sensations

We have talked of 'the same sensation' and 'the same pain', but these phrases always need to be filled out. To be told that this is 'the same pain' tells us nothing unless we are aware of the context. Clearly we have to be told what it is being identified with. It may be the same pain as I had yesterday or half-an-hour ago, or it could be the same pain as I remember when I was a child. Is the phrase being used with the same sense in each of these cases? When we compare the identification of sensations and the identification of my present visual experience with the one I have when I see a London bus, we are clearly thinking of the content of the experience. In this sense of 'same sensation' I group certain sensations together because of some similarity between them, and say that they are the same. We presumably do not group them because of any minor point of likeness, but because they hold their most distinctive feature in common. In the classification of sensations as pains, this is what we have termed 'pain-quality'.

A sensation may have this feature which prompts us to call it a pain, and thus to class it with other similar sensations, but it need not be indistinguishable from other pains. We do draw on imagery from the external world to describe species in the genus 'pain'. 'Stabbing pains' may be instantly recognized as being in some way different from 'pricking pains' or 'shooting pains' and this may have nothing to do with any possible reference to causes. Pricking pains may be very like pains caused by a prick, but not all pricking pains *are* caused by one. A pricking pain is a pain we class with those produced in a certain way, but it is their quality, not their cause, which interests us. 'Shooting pains' with their imagery of shooting stars show this more clearly. It is something intrinsic to the pain, not its cause, which makes us resort to the classification. However, some of these descriptions do have as much of a reference to the intensity as to any quality of the pain. Shooting pains typically leap to a high degree of intensity with a monotonous rhythm. They demand our attention, relax their hold on it, and demand it again with a speedy regularity.

There is, then, a difference of quality, which is expressed in our various classifications, present even in sensations which we judge to be similar in such an important respect that we give them the same name. This might suggest that it is perfectly conceivable for different languages to have their classification of sensations based on different similarities. It would be possible to consider that the differences between the different types of pain were more important than their similarity. The English language makes one feature (i.e. 'pain-quality') the important characteristic, but other languages could have very different assumptions, and even class sensations together because of similarities which English does not recognize. It is, however, reasonable to expect that different languages would by and large recognize the same basic distinctions. It would be strange if Englishmen and, say, Frenchmen did not notice the same features in sensations, particularly if 'pain-quality' is indeed as distinctive an element in sensations as redness is in physical objects.

A sensation must have a quality, just as a thought must have a content, and there is a certain parallel between the quality of pain and the content of a thought. If I claim to have the same thought every time I see a certain modern building, I do not mean that I have the same feeling in my stomach, the same frown on my brow, or the same scowl, or that the thought had the same cause. Neither my reactions nor any cause are sufficient to identify my thought. My thought is not something different from what I think, and when I identify two thoughts which have occurred at separate times, I am saying that I thought the same thing on those occasions. The content of my thought was the same. If I had put into words what I was thinking each time, I would have said exactly the same. Whenever I pass the modern building, I could think how hideous it was. The content of the thought ('What a hideous building') would be the criterion by which to judge whether my thought on the next occasion I passed it was exactly the same. If I then thought that I would like to blow the building up, I could not be said to be having the same thought, even though the cause remained the same. Its content was different. In a similar way the quality of pain provides the criterion for the sameness of pain. A sensation without it could not be termed a pain. It difference in quality means that it is a different sensation. It would be self-contradictory to claim to feel the same sensation and yet to say that it was not a pain now, although it had been one. Similarly one cannot suddenly claim that a certain sensation has now become a pain and yet is still the same sensation. It may be in the same place, and there may have been no perceptible break between one sensation and another, but if one indicates that the sensation now has 'pain-quality' by applying the name 'pain' to it, then the sensation has changed.

G. N. A. Vesey makes a mistake over this. He allows that someone could say of different sensations[1]: 'Yes, I see what they have in common. In a certain respect they did feel the same, although, of course one was a pinching pain, one a cutting pain, and one a burning pain.' Anyone who said this would be recognizing the pain-quality as the most distinctive feature of the sensations, and hence as the ground for classification. To be a 'pain', a sensation would have to 'feel the same' as other pains. It would have to have pain-quality. If it did not, it would not 'feel the same' and would not be called a 'pain'. It would be a different sensation. Vesey is so far implicitly in agreement with the thesis that pain-quality is as much the defining feature of a pain as the content of a thought is of a thought.

Vesey goes on, however, to say[2]: 'There are some sensations which we apprehend as painful under normal conditions, but which under abnormal conditions—say of emotional excitement—we actually welcome. We recognize the sensation as being the same as we would normally find painful, but we no longer find it painful.' If he was just using 'painful' to mean 'unpleasant' there would be no problem. He would be merely claiming that we can sometimes like sensations which we normally dislike. His aim, however, is to show more than that. He is enlarging on a denial he makes that there is a 'merely accidental' connection between pain-quality (or, as he says, the 'feel' of pain) and our reaction to it. He wishes to emphasize that the two march together. It looks as if he is maintaining that, in instances where we welcome sensations pain-quality is no longer present, even if they are the kind of sensations

[1] *The Embodied Mind*, p. 89. [2] op. cit. p. 90.

7

which usually possess it. The sensation is still 'the same', but we no longer recognize it as being a pain, and hence no longer dislike it. This makes the 'feel' of pain a very minor matter, despite the fact that according to Vesey its presence or absence determines whether we like or dislike the sensation. Vesey does not here appear to think it sufficiently important to affect the question whether the sensation is the same or not, and yet he has already quite rightly made it the ground of classifying disparate sensations as 'pains'. Despite their dissimilarities they hold their most distinctive feature in common, and this is why we group them together by giving them the same name. If they lose this feature, and we stop calling them 'pains', they have already changed in their most important respect. A sensation which has lost its outstanding quality can hardly be called 'the same' as it was while it still possessed it. Vesey wants to have it both ways. He denies that the reaction to pain is its defining feature, and talks of the 'feel of pain', which he obviously considers is the basis for our classification of different sensations as pain. At the same time, he appears to think that this defining feature of pain must disappear when we begin to welcome the sensation, instead of trying to avoid it. He claims that it is 'a synthetic proposition' that we have an avoidance reaction to pain, and yet the connection between the two is not 'merely accidental'. There is clearly a tension here.

Vesey must make up his mind. If pains are merely sensations we dislike, then certainly the fact that we no longer find a sensation painful is no guarantee that the sensation has changed. It could be logically possible for it to be 'the same sensation'. I would in that case classify it with the same sensations after my change of attitude as I did before. The fact that I no longer disliked it would mean that I would no longer call it a 'pain', but it would still be 'the same sensation' as I get on other specific occasions, and I could easily give that kind of sensation a particular name. By talking of the 'feel' of pain, Vesey has denied himself this approach. Pains are sensations with a certain quality, and the fact that we usually dislike them is an additional point. The logical consequence of this, however, is that if a sensation no longer possesses that quality, it cannot be called a 'pain', and in fact is a different sensation. It logically cannot be 'the same as we would normally find painful'.

3. *Numerical and Qualitative Identity*

Just as there are other colours besides red, and an object which is not red is not necessarily colourless, so there are other qualities in sensations besides that of pain (although they may not be so distinctive). There are other ways of grouping sensations together. Can we press the parallel further? An object can change colour and still be the same object. Could a sensation change its quality and still be the same sensation? All that we have said so far would suggest not. There is certainly a use of the phrase 'same sensation' which refers exclusively to the quality. When Vesey talked of recognizing the sensation as being the same, he was clearly talking of its 'feel'. If I claim to be feeling the same sensation now as when I broke my leg five years ago, I can hardly be talking about anything except how its feels to me, unless I am saying that my leg has never healed, and I have been in continuous pain. Usually, however, a comparison between two sensations which occurred at widely separate times is a comparison between their qualities. If I claim that I have the same headache now as I did half-an-hour ago, the position is not so clear. Do I merely mean that it has the same quality? In that case I could substitute the words 'exactly similar' for 'the same' without any marked change of sense. I could on the other hand mean that it is numerically the same; I may have felt it continuously for the half-hour, and it may not have changed its position. This would suggest that we do have means of identifying our sensations apart from their quality. It is this fact which enables us to say that '*the* sensation has changed its quality', without necessarily implying that it is a new sensation. It is perhaps significant that such a change would have to be gradual, so that at no one moment could I claim that the sensation had just changed. If a sensation, for example, suddenly acquired a distinctive quality, such as pain-quality, we would normally say that we had a fresh sensation in the same place as the previous one.

The application of different predicates to the same subject demonstrates the importance of numerical identity. It is self-contradictory to say that the pain which I had in my chest today was intolerable, but that at the same time it was bearable, whereas it is not at all self-contradictory to assert that the pain which I had in my chest was intolerable, but that the pain which I had in my arm at the same time was bearable. The difference clearly lies in the fact that in the first case we are talking about one pain, and in the second we are referring to different pains. The predicates do not therefore contradict each other in the second instance, but they do in the first. If we are not clear about what constitutes numerical identity we shall not be clear as to whether we are contradicting ourselves in the application of different predicates. We shall not know whether we are talking about the same sensation or not.

Some sort of continuity in place or time is clearly essential for asserting any numerical identity between sensations. If sensation 'a' at time t_1 is to be regarded as the same as sensation 'b' at time t_2, we must see if the sensation has continued to be felt from t_1 to t_2. Similarly, we must see if 'a' and 'b' were each in the same place, or if they are not, we must ask whether there was a gradual change of position, or if the sensation suddenly appeared to jump from one place to another. If that happened, we could hardly talk of 'a' and 'b' being the same sensation, even if there was some sort of temporal continuity. We might admit, when a sensation had moved slowly and almost imperceptibly up my arm, that sensation 'b' in my shoulder was the same sensation which had been in my wrist, although here we may be partly relying on the qualitative identity of the two sensations. If the sensation had also changed quality slowly, while gradually changing its position, would we be willing to claim that 'b' was numerically identical with 'a'? It would certainly not feel the same, as we could hardly give both sensations the same name. What if a tickle had turned into a pain? We could certainly say that 'the sensation in our wrist' has changed from being a tickle to being a pain. There spatio-temporal continuity enables us to think of the tickle and the pain as being 'the same sensation' (i.e. the sensation in our wrist). A change in position, however gradual, would remove one of the props on which we rest our identification. To claim that the pain in my shoulder is the same sensation as the tickle I previously had in my wrist is uninformative, to say the least. The one may have grown into the other, but apart from this they have nothing in common. They are not qualitatively similar, so I do not have that ground for saying that they are the same. Mere continuity in time, therefore, seems hardly a sufficient ground of identification.

It may be a necessary condition, but in addition we need an identity of place or quality. We can ascribe numerical identity to sensations 'a' and 'b', when they are in the same place but are of different quality, or are of the same quality in a different place, as long as there is temporal continuity, and any change has been gradual. There is, however, no numerical identity which we can ascribe to sensations which occur at different times in the same place, in the way that we have seen the qualitative identity can be ascribed to sensations which occur at different times (and places). Even talk of an intermittent pain in one place would have to rely on the criterion of qualitative identity. Otherwise we would tend to think of a series of pains in the one place rather than the same pain occurring at intervals.

We cannot talk of the identity of sensation 'a' and sensation 'b' unless we have individuated 'a' and 'b' in the first place. Clearly one way by which we refer to sensations is to mention their cause. As we have seen, some descriptions of pain, such as 'pricking', carry a reference to a cause, suggesting that even if this particular pain has not been produced by a prick, it is the kind of pain that is. We use the cause as a means of describing a particular quality of the sensation by linking it in some way to the external world. Would this justify us in assuming that a similarity or identity between the causes of sensations 'a' and 'b' entailed some identity between the sensations? Certainly the same causes tend to bring about the same kind of sensations at different times. This must, however, be an empiricial point and not a logical one. The experience of those who are apparently insensitive to pain, and the possibility of anaesthesia, would suggest that an identical cause might on different occasions or with different people have varying effects. The same cause could produce pain in one person, a sensation which was not recognized as pain in another, and no sensation at all in a third. The possible cause of a sensation cannot therefore be a very good guide for individuating sensations. Because the same cause often does have similar effects, causes are useful as a rough and ready way of describing qualities. If I talk of the kind of sensation I get when such-and-such happens, and suggest that my present sensation is like that, I may be able to give some idea of the kind of sensations with which I would classify what I now feel, and hence some idea of its quality. Cause and sensation are however logically distinct. I can have one without the other, and I do not individuate my sensation by means of the cause. Just because I may find it convenient to refer to the cause, as a means of description, I do not have to look at the cause to decide what kind of sensation I am feeling, or indeed if I am feeling one at all. Similarly if I see something inflicted on someone, which is a normal cause of a particular kind of sensation, I cannot with complete confidence forestall him in talking about his sensation.

Causes are not going to be very helpful as additional criteria of identity. We are left with our distinction between qualitative and numerical identity—the difference between a man when he says that he is now feeling the same pain as he did twenty years ago, but has not been in continuous pain all that time, and when he says that he has the same pain as he did an hour previously, having been in continuous pain. We have seen that numerical identity itself depends on some kind of continuity of quality and position, with the need for temporal continuity thrown in. Do the criteria for each type of identity apply whenever we talk about sensations? Might our manner of reference perhaps already prejudge the question which type of identity is in question? It seems clear that we do have words which describe *episodes* of pain, and only numerical identity could be applicable. A 'stab' of pain must refer to a very short-lived pain, and if we talked of a stab being the same at distinct times, we could only conclude that time t_2 closely followed on time t_1, and that the stab had been a continuous one. We would not assume that they might just be qualitatively identical with no spatio-temporal continuity. If that was so, we would have talked of 'a stab of the same pain' rather than 'the same stab of pain'. In the same way, 'an attack of the same pain' merely refers to an identity of quality, while 'the same attack of pain' could only be an assertion of numerical identity. Twinges and pangs are also brief episodes of pain, or some other type of sensation. I cannot have the same twinge now as I had last week, although here again I could have a twinge of the same pain.

In his book *Attention*[1] A. R. White suggests a rather different

[1] pp. 35–36.

ambiguity in the word 'pain'. He thinks that there is an important distinction to be made between stabs and pangs of pain, and other similar momentary feelings, and what he calls 'continuous discomforts'. The latter are various brands of aches and pains, which are somewhat protracted, such as headaches and pains in the back. His motive for introducing the distinction is a desire to deal with conceptual difficulties which arise over forgetting a pain, because, for example, we are distracted. When we become aware of it again, are we aware of the same feeling as we had before? Is there any sense in saying that we have had it all along, even when we were unaware of it? It certainly seems natural to talk of having the same headache as I had half-an-hour ago, even if I have forgotten about it for most of that time. Clearly we are talking of numerical identity. We do not just mean that my present headache *feels* the same as the one I had half-an-hour ago. We want to say that it *is* the same. This suggests, however, a spatio-temporal continuity for the sensation even when I was unaware of it, and we are faced with the possibility of unfelt sensations (which we have denied in previous chapters). Examples of forgetting pains, however, as opposed to their simply stopping for a time, logically, depend on some kind of distraction. I may forget my headache because I am interested in an argument which I am having with someone. If my interest in the argument flags, I will remember my headache. If I do not, then I would be under no temptation to say that I still had it. An 'unfelt sensation' must be regarded as a contradiction, but we are justified in talking about forgetting sensations and then feeling the *same* one after a gap, when we would have felt them if we had not been distracted. If I forget the pain from a blister because of my absorption in a game, my only grounds for talking of 'forgetting' it, and for not saying that it had gone, would be that I felt it again the minute my concentration on the game gave way. I could say that I would have felt it but for my absorption, and this gives us ground for thinking of some kind of continuity. It is however a logical continuity, rather than that of some shadowy pain which is 'there' in some way, but just happens not to be felt.

We must return to White's method of dealing with this problem. He does not stress the logical importance of distraction as we have done. He uses his distinction between stabs of pain and continuous pains, and suggests that continuous pains are constituted by a series (which may be broken) of stabs or twinges. This enables him to say[1]: 'What we notice or fail to notice in continuous feelings like discomforts are the momentary feelings, like stabs, twinges, throbs or pangs, which are their signs.' What White, misleadingly, calls 'discomforts' are supposed to have a dispositional sense, so that we can talk of having a pain, even when we do not actually feel anything. What we mean is that we are liable to feel stabs or twinges (and White thinks that we cannot have these unfelt). He can thus say: 'A man with a present headache feels and is liable to feel intermittent stabs of pain.' He also claims: 'In a present headache the gaps are void of any twinges or throbs.' This dispositional sense of 'headache' and 'pain' certainly helps him in dealing with the problem which he sets himself of forgetting feelings. It means that we can quite cheerfully say that we forgot our headache or pain, without worrying about the fact that this implies that it still existed in some way. Our disposition to have stabs still did exist. We just did not have any for a certain period of time.

This theory certainly seems to deal in a neat way with the problem it was designed to meet, but that is its only virtue. Apart from the special case of distraction, when we say that we have or had a pain we mean that we could feel it. If I claim to have had a headache for the whole afternoon, I mean that I had a diffuse dull pain which was continuous. I do not mean that I had a series of 'intermittent stabs of pain'. A series of stabs of pain would certainly not be an ache. It would be a completely different species of pain. In fact it would not be counted one pain at all. The stabs may be all stabs of the same kind of pain, but they would be distinct numerically. A series of stabs is different from a stabbing pain. The stabbing pain may consist of stabs of pain, but the difference is that although the pain may come to be of greater intensity for brief moments, there is not a pause when no pain can be felt. There is a substratum of pain of lower intensity present even when the pain is not actually stabbing.

White tries to solve the difficulty raised by a pain which we want to say is numerically the same as one we felt before we were distracted despite a temporal break. He does it by taking

[1] *Attention* p. 35.

the difficulty of one particular type of situation and generalizing it, so that it crops up in any stretch of continuous pain. Just as we hesitate about asserting numerical identity of a pain which apparently stops or is not felt for a while, so we must hesitate about asserting numerical identity of continuous pains which in fact turn out to be merely a series of stabs or twinges. A 'present headache' is a continuous ache which I have at the moment in my head. It should not be a succession of twinges or throbs with gaps between them, when I feel no pain. If the latter were the case, I would more naturally talk of having *pains* in my head instead of one pain or ache. Rather than dismiss temporal continuity as a necessary condition of identity, White would have done better to try to extend the concept of such continuity in some way, so as to cover cases of distraction. As we have already said, the fact that we would have felt the pain if we had not been distracted, is surely sufficient to provide the idea of a kind of continuity.

White appears to think that anxiety should be treated in the same way as pain. Just as someone with a headache has intermittent stabs of pain, he says[1]: 'Someone who is now anxious feels and is liable to feel pangs of anxiety'. He supposes that if we forget a headache, we do not feel any stabs of pain, and if we forget our anxiety we do not feel any unpleasant pangs. Although anxiety is normally an emotion and headache a sensation, White treats them both as if they were parallel in every way. He appears to ignore the fact that we are normally anxious about something, whereas we never have a headache *at* anything. In other words he ignores the point that emotions typically take 'objects'. He seems to think that anxiety is as much a matter of merely having 'pangs' as a headache is of feeling pain. In what appears to be a definition he says: 'To have a present headache or to be now anxious is to suffer from and be liable to occasional, frequent, or even a continuous series of stabs of pain and pangs of anxiety.' Clearly there must be more to it than this. How could we say that we felt pangs of *anxiety*, if the pangs were all that there were to anxiety? White, of course, could envisage pangs which had a distinctive 'anxiety-quality'. When I had them I would know I was anxious. If I did not, then either I was not anxious, or I had forgotten my anxiety.

[1] op. cit. p. 35.

However the main difference between a pang of anxiety, a pang of fear, a pang of disappointment, or a pang of any other emotion, would seem to be their contexts. It is because they occur in certain situations that I attribute them to various emotions. A pang of anxiety, for instance, would occur in a situation which I viewed as disquieting in some way. We have already seen how it is possible to be anxious about the significance of a pain, because one thinks it is the sign of the onslaught of a fatal disease. Such anxiety would be defined by our belief about the pain, and not by any pang which might occur apart from the pain. Indeed even if I felt no special pangs, I might still be said to be anxious. If pangs which I recognized as being like those I might feel when anxious occurred when, for example, I had just received news of some personal failure when I had hoped for success, I would not have to say that I was anxious and not disappointed. The situation was one of disappointment, and the pangs would be called pangs of disappointment, whether they were similar or not to pangs of anxiety. This is all in marked contrast to stabs of pain, which are stabs of pain, if they are recognized as such, whatever their context.

4. *The Identity of Emotions*

We cannot use the same kind of criteria for the identity of emotions, as we do for that of sensations. Any pangs I may have in a situation are completely irrelevant to the question whether my present anxiety is the same as the one I had yesterday or ten years ago. There are not different species of pangs, within the genus of those with 'anxiety-quality', to tell us whether this anxiety is the same as that. I must compare the 'objects' of my anxiety in each instance. I may have been anxious last week about an examination at the end of the week, and have been worried about whether I would be able to answer the questions, but now that I have taken the examination I could hardly be anxious about the same thing. What I was worried about is over; I may certainly now be anxious about the results, but this is a different anxiety. Similarly, if I talk of having the same fear as I used to have or as everybody else admits to having, this does not mean that the same kind of pangs are present. It means that we are afraid of the same thing. Different people who are afraid of the dark could all be said to have the same fear.

Temporal continuity is not as important for the identity of emotions as for that of sensations. To be said to have the same fear as yesterday, I need not have been continuously afraid for the whole of the intervening period. I need only be afraid of the same thing. This, and the irrelevance of any bodily feelings we may have for any question of identity, indicates that we cannot apply the notions of numerical and qualitative identity to emotions, as we did to sensations. There is instead a distinction to be made between an 'object' being *the same* as the 'object' of a possibly different emotion, and it being *similar* in an important respect. The difference is between talking of two emotional episodes being instances of the same fear, and saying that they are both instances of *fear*, as opposed to any other emotion. In both cases we could talk of 'the same emotion'. In the first we could mean that it was exactly the same, that it had an identical 'object' as the other instance. In the second, we would mean that both instances were examples of the same kind of emotion, that the 'objects' had enough in common for us to classify them together. I could be said to have the same fear if I was afraid of a particular kind of danger on different occasions. My emotion on each occasion would then be the same. If, on the other hand, I was in an agitated or disturbed state, when faced with different kinds of danger, I could be said to be afraid on each occasion. Again I would be said to have the same emotion. In the one case, the implied contrast would be with other kinds of fear (i.e. fear with different kinds of 'objects'); in the other, it would be with other kinds of emotion apart from fear. As phrases like 'the same fear' or 'the same jealousy' mark one kind of fear or jealousy off from different kinds very effectively, we would expect any mention of 'the same emotion' to be usually intended to distinguish between different kinds of emotion, rather than different brands of the same emotion. To ask whether this was the same emotion as that, rather than merely the same fear, would be to ask whether the 'objects' have enough in common for us to be able to claim that the view of the situation was the same in a major respect, even though the details of each situation were very different. If, for example, we viewed each situation as dangerous, we would be justified in using the word 'fear' of both, and thus in classing them together as the same emotion. However different a nation's imperialism may be from a bull charging at me, I could justly be said to be afraid of both, if I thought that the imperialism was as much of a menace to my interests (interpreted in the widest possible sense) as the bull in its way.

All this is clearly relevant to problems that have arisen in previous chapters. If the emotion which as we have argued, is, usually present in an experience of physical pain, is the same as or very similar to, the emotion of mental pain or distress, we would expect our view of both types of situation to be similar in an important respect. By talking of distress in connection with physical pain we have deliberately implied that the same emotion is present both in mental pain and in normal cases of physical pain. By associating dislike and distress and by suggesting that the one grows into the other, at least when physical pain is the 'object', we have implied that dislike (when an emotion) and distress are very similar. Clearly the only way to decide if claims like these are correct is to decide how similar our views of the various situations are.

A typical situation of mental pain is one of bereavement. Whether I said that a bereavement was 'very painful' or 'very distressing' would be immaterial. In such situations 'pain' and 'distress' are more or less synonymous. How, then, does bereavement compare with an unbearable physical pain, as an 'object' of distress? Certainly I could talk of being very distressed at the pain, but even if I did not use the word and instead talked merely of 'agony', we might ask if distress is normally involved. Am I experiencing the same emotion? Situations of distress are typically ones which I dislike very much, which I find very unpleasant, and from which I would like to be extricated. Very often, however, I am powerless to do anything about it. An animal 'in distress' may be completely helpless. If I am distressed at a bereavement, I may profoundly wish that it had not happened, but there is nothing I can do about it. I may weep and moan helplessly or I may sternly try to repress my inclination to do so, but I cannot alter the situation. Clearly my attitude to physical pain is almost identical. It is something I profoundly dislike. There may be something I could do in an indirect way to be rid of the pain, unlike a bereavement, but all too often it may be something I just have to endure for a short or long time. Distress is an emotional reaction to situations which I regard as being very bad and unpleasant for me in some way. I may wish to be rid of the situation or the sensation, or I may be merely left wishing that it had never happened. My attitude in situations which I dislike may be less emphatic, but it is obviously similar. I may merely prefer to be without whatever it is I dislike, but I still regard it as unpleasant. It is significant that in trying to put into words our typical view of 'objects' of distress we had to use phrases such as 'profoundly dislike'. I just take an even more adverse view of the situation when I am distressed by it than when I dislike it. It matters very little whether the situation is of something like bereavement or of physical pain. Our attitude to each is so nearly identical that we can plausibly claim to be feeling the same emotion in each case.

VI

IS PLEASURE A SENSATION?

1. *Sensations of Pleasure*

PHILOSOPHERS have been regularly tempted to think of pain in terms of displeasure because of their desire to treat the concepts of pain and pleasure in the same way. For the same reason, some philosophers have readily assumed that if pain is a sensation, pleasure must be as well. Bentham is an obvious example of someone who thought that all pleasure and all pain should be analysed on the lines of physical pain.

In the light of our discussion of pain, we must now question whether the concepts of pain and pleasure are similar. In particular, we must ask whether there is a class of sensations of pleasure which we form because of our recognition of a certain similarity between the different sensations. It is not enough to say that there is no similarity, but that it is just a fact that we do group those particular sensations together. There must be some basis for our classification, to explain our ability to cope with new instances. We are able to say quite definitely, without examining our reaction or the situation, whether a new species of sensation is a pain or not. Can we do the same with pleasure? Can we decide whether a sensation is one of pleasure merely from its quality? We have seen that the concept of discomfort does not allow us to prise the sensation away from the reaction in this way. Is there a pleasure-quality, or are sensations of pleasure grouped, like these sensations, solely on the basis of our reaction to them?

To talk legitimately of a pleasure-quality it need not be the case that *all* pleasure involves feeling a distinctive type of sensation. We would expect to make the same kind of distinction between mental and physical pleasure as we have made between mental and physical pain. The main difference between the two types of pleasure may merely lie in the kind of 'object', but, from wherever it stems, pleasure-quality would only be associated with physical pleasure. It would be the quality of a sensation, and of nothing else. In terms of the definition of a sensation, which we have assumed throughout, it would be the quality of a feeling which can be definitely located in the body, and which has a distinct beginning and end.

We would not expect pleasure-quality to be linked with mental pleasure, any more than pain-quality is involved in distress and other forms of mental pain. It may be suggested that we do feel thrills of pleasure in situations where our pleasure might be described as 'mental', and where the 'object' of our pleasure need not be a sensation. Could these thrills have pleasure-quality? It might certainly be plausible to call such feelings 'sensations'. The fact that they may be more pervasive than many sensations of pain, for example, does not mean that they are not locatable. There is an answer to the question as to where we feel them even if it is merely 'all over'. A sensation of cold in my arm does not stop being a sensation when it spreads over the body. Just as we can locate it, we can time it as well as any other sensation. It would have a beginning and an end.

Do we say that these thrills are thrills of pleasure, because they feel the same and we group them together as having some quality in common? It is completely wrong to compare thrills of pleasure with sensations of pain and other sensations which we group together because of their quality. What thrills of pleasure have in common is their context. They may or may not feel similar to each other, and distinctive from other thrills. They might even feel exactly the same as, say, a thrill of fear. This could be our ground for giving the name 'thrill' to both feelings. All this, however, is irrelevant to their being thrills *of pleasure*. They are that because of their context. We would never claim to recognize a thrill of pleasure in a situation where we deny being pleased about anything. It is unintelligible to claim to be thoroughly miserable and discontented with everything, and yet to say that nevertheless the situation is brightened by the fact that one is feeling a thrill of pleasure. This is very much in contrast with pain. It is by no means odd to say that one is overjoyed at some situation, but that the whole thing is slightly marred by the fact that one is in physical pain. Thrills of pleasure need not be themselves pleasant, since what is pleasant is the situation in which they occur. They are to be compared not with sensations of pain (which are normally painful) but with thrills of fear or feelings of anger. The latter are not themselves frightening or irritating. They merely occur in situations where we are frightened or angry at something else.

Thrills of pleasure are not candidates as sensations with pleasure-quality, which could be compared with sensations of pain. They were never, however, the main contenders. When it is suggested that the concepts of pain and pleasure are parallel, it is usually supposed that there are sensations of pleasure which, like those of pain, are recognized as such without regard to their context. They would have a distinctive quality, and that would be our reason for talking of 'pleasure'. After we have learnt the concept, the situation in which such sensations occur would be as irrelevant to deciding what kind of sensations they are as are the situations in which we feel pain, although we would expect a normal link with a particular kind of reaction. If there is a concept of pleasure-quality lurking in our assumptions about pleasure, and if it functions like pain-quality, it would be logically possible to feel a sensation of pleasure and not like it. It would even be intelligible if we completely disliked it. We would recognize that the sensation was similar in a most important respect to other sensations which we normally liked, and for that reason we would be impelled to call it 'pleassure', and hence acknowledge our inclination to classify it with those sensations. Nevertheless our reaction to the sensation would not be a normal one. If the parallel is to be maintained, it should also be possible to like a sensation very much, and even take (mental) pleasure in it, and yet deny that it was in any way a sensation of pleasure because it had no distinctive quality. We would thus have to drive a logical wedge between a 'pleasant sensation' (merely a sensation which is liked) and a 'sensation of pleasure', in the same way as we have distinguished between an unpleasant or distressing sensation and a sensation of pain.

Not all unpleasant sensations are sensations of pain, so we must expect to find some pleasant sensations which are not sensations of pleasure. If, however, the two concepts are parallel, very many pleasant sensations should have something in common apart from the fact that they are liked. If they do not share in any such similarity, we must conclude that there is no such concept as that of pleasure-quality. Any likeness of the kind we are interested in would be the main ground of our liking for the sensation and, if it disappeared, the sensation would have changed in its most important respect. It would probably not even be pleasant any longer.

We have agreed that, even if there are sensations of pleasure, *all* pleasure need not involve sensations and all pleasant sensations need not be sensations of pleasure. This, however, contradicts two assumptions that are often made by philosophers in discussing whether pleasure is a sensation. They appear to think that if they can show that pleasant sensations are not involved in some experiences of pleasure, and that sensations can be pleasant without having any distinctive quality of pleasure, then they have demonstrated that pleasure is not a sensation. They have not in fact proved more than that, if there is a pleasure-quality, it is only one part of the concept of pleasure. A. R. White,[1] for example, seems to think that he has denied that pleasure is a sensation by pointing out that a child who immensely enjoys a circus is not 'merely or mainly the recipient of pleasant sensations'. He has certainly shown that, if there is a pleasure-quality, it cannot be used to explain every instance of pleasure, but he thinks that he has done more than that. Similarly he says: 'Bodily sensations, such as the feel of soft fur on the skin . . . can be very pleasant. But this does not make pleasure a sensation.' Here he has shown that pleasure-quality need not be involved even when we are taking pleasure in a sensation. The feel of soft fur on the skin is a sensation we may like, but it is hard to see that it has anything in common with other types of sensation which we like, apart from the fact that we like them. Again, however, White has not proved as much as he thinks. He has shown that not all sensations which we like are sensations of pleasure. He has not shown that none are.

There is a tendency for experimental psychologists to assume that if a sensation is sought after, it must be one of pleasure. This is largely because of their desire to give a behavioural definition of pleasure. In some experiments electrodes are implanted in the brains of animals and a circuit is arranged so that

[1] *Attention*, p. 111.

animals can give themselves a shock. It is reported that when electrodes are in certain places animals stimulate their brains more than five thousand times an hour.[1] It is sometimes claimed that this shows that there are 'pleasure centres' in the brain, the stimulation of which gives feelings of pleasure. It need show no such thing, even if the animals are feeling something. The fact that the animals seek out the shocks might suggest that they get sensations they like from them. In other words, they receive pleasant sensations. The experiments do not (and could not) prove that they feel sensations of pleasure.

Many philosophers do not make this distinction between pleasant sensations and sensations of pleasure. As a result they tend to assume that if they can indicate bodily sensations which give pleasure, they have shown that there are sensations of pleasure and that these are the opposite of pain. They do not realize that to take pleasure in a sensation is merely to find the sensation pleasant, and nothing follows as to whether the sensation has a special quality which gives the pleasure. We shall mention, in connection with masochism, Hospers's distinction between pleasure as the opposite of displeasure and the pleasure which is derived from bodily sensations and is the opposite of pain. He says[2]: 'There are pleasurable sensations, such as those of being tickled, stroked and rubbed; since these pleasures have a definite bodily location, here it makes sense to ask *"Where* do you feel the pleasure?".' He compares this with asking where a pain is felt, and concludes that this type of pleasure is the 'opposite' of physical pain. If pain is not merely a sensation which is disliked, this parallel cannot necessarily be upheld. Hospers has given examples of sensations we like and take pleasure in, but he has not suggested that they have any quality in common which might function like pain-quality. Is it significant that we can talk of 'pleasures', and not just pleasant sensations'? Certainly a question such as 'Where do you feel pleasure?' seems to be the same kind of question as, 'Where do you feel pain?', although it is a far less common thing to say. Whether it need be anything more than a request for the location of a sensation we like is doubtful. I can have many pleasures

[1] See 'Self-Stimulation Experiments and Differentiated Reward Systems' by J. Olds, reprinted in *Motivation*, Penguin Modern Psychology, p. 297.

[2] *Human Conduct*, p. 112.

in my life, but like sailing or motoring they are merely the things which I enjoy or take pleasure in. They need have nothing in common besides that. Need the use of the word 'pleasure' in connection with sensations suggest anything different?

The pleasurable sensations to which Hospers refers could, from what he says, be merely pleasant sensations. As they are sensations, it clearly makes sense to ask where we feel them. They may still be sensations which we take pleasure in, and not sensations of pleasure which hold a distinctive quality in common. W. B. Gallie[1] also appears to assume that he has only to refer to sensations which can be called 'pleasures' to show that some pleasure is as much a special class of sensation as physical pain. He says:

Think of such instances as the following: at the end of the closed season a man feels again a rifle or a cricket-bat in his hands: a woman takes an infant into her arms: chilled through and through, we put our feet on a hot-water bottle. Are not such pleasures anyhow roughly clockable and locatable?

We can certainly time and locate the feelings which Gallie mentions. To take the force of the examples we must assume that we take pleasure in the sensations themselves, and not in any significance which they may have. We may for example relish the fact that the feel of the cricket-bat is a sign that the new season is beginning, and not be particularly enamoured of the sensation for its own sake. Even if the sensations themselves give us pleasure, we are still nowhere near the concept of pleasure-quality. Has the feel of a cricket-bat anything in common with the feel of an infant, or that of a hot-water bottle when we put our chilled feet on it? It seems ridiculous even to pose the question, and yet it is not ridiculous to ask whether, for instance, stabbing pains and burning pains have anything in common. Gallie's examples of 'pleasure' cannot be examples of a genus of sensations, as individual pains are examples of the genus 'pain'. The only thing which they can have in common is our attitude to them and our reaction in general. They are feelings which give us pleasure, in the sense that we like them, and this alone gives us the justification for calling them

---

[1] *Proceedings of the Aristotelian Society, Supplementary Volume*, xxviii (1954), 148.

'pleasure'. The pleasure which we derive from the feel of a cricket-bat does not come because the sensation has a special quality which prompts us to compare it with the feel of a hot-water bottle. It is a matter of our attitude to the sensation. If our attitude to it changed, as it might by the end of a long innings when our arms were aching, we would be under no possible temptation to say that we are still feeling a sensation of pleasure, but that we no longer like it.

It might be suggested that Gallie's case is weakened by his choice of examples, some of which are hardly central cases of physical pleasure. If we were to compare feeling a hot-water bottle when chilled with the delight of a cool hand on a hot head, would we be any nearer finding a pleasure-quality? Even if on a particular occasion we liked neither sensation, could we say that in each case we were feeling the same sensation? Both can undoubtedly be physical pleasures. Might we feel a completely new type of pleasant sensation and recognize that it was in an important respect like these sensations and thus a sensation of pleasure? Could we compare them to sexual sensations and group them all together as 'the same sensation', without suggesting they were all sexual or all possessed qualities of warmth or coolness? If there were sensations of pleasure on the model of sensations of pain, the answer to all these questions would be 'yes', and this seems implausible.

If there is a pleasure-quality, we could envisage having sensations which changed suddenly in one respect. They would become sensations of pleasure, whereas previously we would not have recognized them as such. Just as a stinging or a pricking sensation can become a stinging or pricking *pain*, so an ordinary sensation of warmth or of coolness could become a pleasure. Just as the new pain need not be disliked, so the new pleasure need not be liked. We can understand someone who says that a sensation has just become a pain, but that he does not dislike it yet. Could we understand anyone who said that his sensation has just become a pleasure, but he doesn't have any more liking for it than he did before? It is significant that it would be more natural for him to say it was now pleasurable, and this certainly entails liking, just as the word 'painful' implies dislike.

The reason we normally dislike a pricking pain is that it is a pain, and not that it is a pricking sensation. If it is maintained that sensations of warmth or coolness have a special quality because they are pleasures, this suggests that we like that quality, and not the warmth or the coolness. It suggests that I like to feel a cool hand on my hot brow because it is a sensation of pleasure, and not because I like the feeling of coolness. I like to feel a hot-water bottle when I am chilled because I like feeling pleasure, and not warmth. It is, however, clear that in these cases it is the warmth and the coolness which we appreciate and nothing else. In the one case we are chilled and want to feel warm, and in the other we are hot and want to feel cool.

If there is a pleasure-quality, pleasant sensations must not be confused with sensations of pleasure. What candidates are left as sensations of pleasure? The obvious one are 'bodily pleasures' connected with elementary bodily functions. Sexual pleasure and the pleasure of eating provide two central examples. Might it be significant how naturally the word 'pleasure' can be used in this connection? Kenny[1] is under no doubt that 'some pleasures are sensations'. He concludes: 'Since pleasure may be a sensation, and pain need not be, pain and pleasure are not perhaps as ill-assorted a pair as they are sometimes said to be.' Although he gives sexual pleasure as an example, and must have something like pleasure-quality in mind, it sometimes seems that Kenny means no more by saying that pleasure may be a sensation than that some types of sensation are pleasant. He says in the same context: 'Though some sensations are pleasant, pleasure is not in general a sensation.'

Kenny attempts to force a comparison between pleasure and pain by saying: 'One may feel pleasure from a caress, as one may feel pain from a blow.' He is trading on an ambiguity in the phrase 'feel pleasure from a caress'. His comparison with blows which cause pain suggests that he is thinking of caresses causally producing a distinctive brand of sensation. It would, however, be more normal to understand it as meaning that we take pleasure in the caress, that we like the sensation it gives us. In other words the caress (or sensation produced by it, as 'caress' like 'touch' is ambiguous) is the 'object', and not necessarily the cause of our pleasure. We have to be aware of it to take pleasure in it, whereas we do not have to be aware of its cause. If we feel pain, we do not have to be aware of the blow which caused it. We

[1] *Action, Emotion and Will*, p. 128.

can therefore be said to be feeling pleasure from x without necessarily assuming, as Kenny appears to, that there is a sensation called pleasure, which x causes. We may be merely finding x pleasant to a greater or lesser degree.

Kenny considers[1] that it is possible to recognize sensations of pain or of pleasure on a particular occasion independently of our attitude towards them, and in doing this he implicitly admits the need for concepts of pain-quality and of pleasure-quality. If our attitude or reaction to a sensation does not govern how we classify it, then we must be relying on its quality. We must be recognizing its similarity to other sensations. How far does his parallel hold between sensations of pain and sexual sensations and other bodily pleasures? One worry which is sometimes raised about talk of such 'pleasures' is, as A. R. Manser[2] says: 'It is as if certain sensations couldn't but be pleasurable.' If the comparison with pain is pressed, it can be readily seen that this difficulty has no substance. Although it would be normal to like a bodily pleasure, and although the concept of pleasure-quality would have to be taught by means of situations where a sensation was obviously liked, there would be no contradiction in denying that a particular sensation of pleasure was liked. It would be no more odd to say that some pleasures were not pleasurable than to say that some pains were not painful. The sensation has been separated from its normal reaction, but that is a perfectly intelligible situation.

It is logically possible for there to be a class of sensations with distinctive quality in common, which are normally liked for that quality. Sexual sensations are often cited as an example, and they certainly are of this type. Is their quality, however, one that could be properly called a 'pleasure-quality'? Can they be classified with other sensations because they have the quality in common with them? So far from having any quality in common, sexual sensations are usually considered to be so distinctive as to form a special class of their own. They are not just one species of a distinctive genus as a stabbing pain is a species of pain. It is very apparent that sexual pleasure has little in common with, say, the pleasures of eating. Both provide sensations which we usually like, but the sensations are

---

[1] *Action, Emotion and Will*, p. 142.
[2] *Proceedings of the Aristotelian Society*, vol lxii (1960–1), 226.

completely dissimilar. To assimilate a pleasant taste to sexual pleasure on the grounds that they both come under the umbrella-concept of 'sensation of pleasure' is clearly ridiculous. Equally implausible would be any attempt to suggest that different tastes had the same quality, and could be classified as being in some way the same sensation, merely because they were pleasant. A pleasant taste is one which we enjoy, and we can enjoy many different tastes, without there being any suggestion that we enjoy the same thing in each of them. Indeed, we may enjoy an unusual taste precisely because it *is* utterly different from other tastes which we might also find pleasant.

If tastes are not sensations of pleasure, could any of the other pleasures of eating be put in that category? What of the feeling of having eaten after a good and satisfying meal? This seems impossible to reduce to specific sensations which we like. It is rather a pervasive feeling of well-being and contentment. There seem to be no distinctive sensations here which could be likened to sexual sensations, and classed as 'sensations of pleasure'. Sexual sensations are often quoted as the paradigm of such sensations, but it is beginning to look as if they are the only possible examples. Although they have a quality which is normally liked, in the same way in which pain-quality is normally disliked, they form a narrow range of sensations which are unique. Are these to be our sensations of pleasure, as a conceptual counterbalance to sensations of pain? If they are, their distinctive quality must be the pleasure-quality we are searching for. In that case all sensations of pleasure will be sexual sensations and vice versa. Our ground for grouping sensations of pleasure together will be identical with our ground for classifying sensations as sexual.

It seems very implausible to suggest that only one type of sensation, from one source, possesses pleasure-quality. Why should we term it 'pleasure-quality', instead of merely accepting that the distinctive quality of sexual sensations is normally liked by most people? In the absence of any point of similarity between such sensations and other pleasant sensations there seems little point in giving sexual sensations a special status. Why should we maintain that those sensations have pleasure-quality any more than other distinctive sensations which most people like? The point of postulating such a quality would be to stress an important similarity which existed between different types of pleasant sensations, and to suggest that they were normally liked because of what they held in common. Stabbing pains and burning pains are normally disliked, and they are largely disliked for the same reason, namely because they have pain-quality. If each type was merely normally unpleasant, and did not share any special similarity apart from that, we would not feel drawn to set up the stabbing quality or the burning quality as a special pain-quality. To do so would be to introduce an unnecessary concept. We would already have the concept of a stabbing or burning quality to explain our grouping of certain sensations together and our recognition of new instances as being similar. Why should we want to set up the quality of one species of pleasant sensation as a special pleasure-quality? Many tickles are pleasant, but it would be very implausible to enthrone sensations which we class as tickles as the only sensations of pleasure. Sexual pleasure is liked more than mere tickles, but that is not sufficient ground for talking about pleasure-quality in connection with it and no other type of pleasant sensation. Our reaction to a sensation is irrelevant to the question as to what kind it is.

We must be content to identify certain sensations as sexual, and not give the same class of sensation a different name as well. The concept of a sensation of pleasure must embrace more than sexual sensations, if it embraces any sensation. If sexual sensations are the only candidates as sensations with pleasure-quality, then we must conclude that the concept of pleasure-quality is superfluous and that the distinction between 'pleasant sensations' and 'sensations of pleasure' is an unreal one. It is logically possible that there is a similarity between different types of pleasant sensations, which could be the reason we normally like them. If there was, our concept of pleasure would include the idea of a 'pleasure-quality', and it would be a different concept from the one we in fact hold.

It might be suggested that even though there was no particular pleasure-quality, there might be several distinctive qualities which would prompt us to say that sensations which possessed them were sensations of pleasure. They could not form a clearly delineated and restricted class, as we have to be able to say whether new instances which we have not met before fall within it or not. The qualities must therefore be merely those which we tend to like, and clearly the quality of sexual sensations would be amongst them. In that case, even though there would be no 'pleasure-quality', as we have used the term, we would be able to talk of a 'sensation of pleasure', even on an occasion when we did not find it pleasant. It would possess a quality which we would recognize as being normally pleasant. In doing so, we would not necessarily be suggesting that it was similar to other species of sensations of pleasure. This analysis would clearly prise apart the concept of sensations of pleasure from that of sensations of pain. A similar treatment of the latter would not be possible, as there are species of sensations, such as those produced by electric shock, which we normally dislike and yet which we deny are pains. On a view like the one we are considering we have no means of saying that such a species was not pain, as pains would be just those kinds of sensations which are normally disliked.

With regard to pleasure we would have no means of saying that a type of sensation which we normally like was not a sensation of pleasure. Does this matter? By saying that a sensation was one of pleasure we would be suggesting that it is to be so regarded even in instances where we do not like it. Even then, however, we would simply mean that the sensation is of a type which is normally liked, even if it is not liked at the moment. As we would not be specifying any one particular type, a sensation of pleasure would merely be a kind of sensation which is normally pleasant. Even if we restricted the term to the sensations which were normally *very* pleasant, the concept of a sensation of pleasure would still be logically dependent on that of a pleasant sensation. If we understood what a pleasant sensation was, we would understand what a sensation of pleasure was, although the two descriptions would not be synonymous. Not all sensations which are sometimes pleasant are normally pleasant, and not all types of sensation which are normally pleasant are always pleasant. We could thus draw a clear distinction between a 'pleasant sensation' and a 'sensation of pleasure', without implying that all 'sensations of pleasure' had any quality in common. The trouble is that this is precisely what seems to be implied by the phrase. It seems to suggest that there is a sensation called 'pleasure', which is different from a mere pleasant sensation, in the same way that 'pain' is a definite sensation and to be distinguished from an 'unpleasant sensation'. It indicates that physical pleasure is to be analysed in the same way as physical pain. For this reason talk of 'sensations of pleasure' is misleading. It is perhaps significant that we do not tend to use the phrase in ordinary situations, and that references to 'physical pleasures' or 'bodily pleasures' more usually occur when we want to talk about sensations which we normally find pleasant.

2. *Pleasantness and Liking*

Just as the unpleasantness of a pain must be distinguished from pain-quality, so the pleasantness of a sensation must not be thought to be a property of the sensation. If there is no pleasure-quality, all that pleasant sensations have in common is their pleasantness. In other words, we like them. If we did not like a sensation, we would not call it 'pleasant', and if we did like it, it must be pleasant. 'Pleasantness' appears to be a feature of the sensation, and to call a sensation 'pleasant' appears to be a remark about the sensation. We must not, however, be misled by grammar. A view may be pleasant, and so may a scent, or some types of weather, but if we say that they are, we are not thereby attributing some special characteristic to them. We are talking primarily about people's reaction to them. We like the view, the scent or the weather. There will of course be reasons why we like them. We may like the view because we like wide-open spaces. We will not however like it because of a special property 'pleasantness' which it possesses.

We know what kind of things most people like, so we may have a good idea what type of weather 'pleasant weather' would be. We would be surprised if someone claimed that heavy rain or icy weather was pleasant. We would not, however, conclude anything about the weather from his remarks. We would assume that he had peculiar tastes. If we maintained that the same weather was unpleasant, would we be contradicting him? Clearly it is merely a matter of our disliking what he likes. We may appeal to other people's likes and dislikes to show that that particular type of weather is normally regarded as unpleasant, and a sense could thus be given to saying that he likes 'unpleasant' weather. This is not to suggest that the unpleasantness of weather consists in anything more than people's attitude to it. There is no one feature which different types of unpleasant weather have in common except that people dislike them. If anyone does not dislike them, then he does not find them unpleasant. If we said that we liked the weather because it was pleasant, we would in fact be giving no reason at all. It would be equivalent to saying, in reply to a question as to why we liked it, 'I just like it, that's all'. In other words, I don't know what it is that I especially like about it. To be really informative I would have to say that I liked the weather because, say, it was dry and warm.

To say that something is pleasant is not to suggest that we gain great pleasure from it. We do not become ecstatic with joy merely through liking something. There are degrees of pleasure. This might appear to support those who want to keep the concepts of pleasure and pain parallel. Are there not degrees of pain? Sensations of pain can be more or less intense. Does not the fact that there are degrees of pleasure show that, at least when we take pleasure in sensations, the pleasure is a quality of the sensations? When they are intense, we feel a large amount of pleasure, and when they are barely noticeable, we only feel a small degree of pleasure. This proposal bears very little examination. Sensations may be intense in a way that emotions are not, but emotions can also be said to have intensity. We can feel degrees of fear or anger. I can be slightly afraid or in a panic. I can be peeved or in a rage. In these cases there can be no suggestion that the growth of intensity consists in sensations becoming more noticeable. My view of the situation is what is important. In fear it can change from one where I think the circumstances embody a slight threat to one in which I am almost overcome by what I conceive as a major threat. My general agitation will increase step by step with the change in my outlook. A change from dislike to distress largely consists in our taking an even more adverse view of the situation we are in. Even if no part of the concept of pleasure balances that of physical pain, it will still be intelligible to talk of degrees of pleasure. If the concept of pleasure is at all similar to the concept of an emotion, we can feel intense pleasure without necessarily having any particular noticeable sensations. Similarly getting mild pleasure need not involve having sensations of any sort. If something gives us a mild degree of pleasure on a particular occasion, we can be said merely to like it. This sense of 'like', which refers to a particular reaction on a particular occasion, must be distinguished from the dispositional sense. I can like this particular meal of roast beef without usually liking roast beef, and I can like roast beef in general without liking this particular meal. When we talk of what we like, we are often using the dispositional sense, and we are talking of what tends to give us pleasure. We might, however, be saying that something is giving us pleasure now, just as it is possible to speak of disliking a pain which I may have now. In other words there are episodes of liking just as there are episodes of disliking.

Not all such episodes have any connection with pleasure. We can be said to like things both in the episodic and dispositional senses, without there being any suggestion that we enjoy them or take pleasure in them. As we said in Chapter III, there are senses of 'like' and 'dislike' with which we can deliver a considered judgement about a situation. When we use them, we are saying that we approve or disapprove of something. If I say that I liked a particular theatrical production, I may mean that I enjoyed it, but I am just as likely to mean that I approved of it or appreciated it. This distinction does not normally apply when we talk of sensations. If we like a sensation, we only mean that we gain some pleasure from it. The context would have to be very peculiar, when we said that we liked a particular sensation, for us to mean that we approved of it.

We have suggested that some episodes of liking are episodes of mild pleasure. To like something can be to find it pleasant, and to find it pleasant is to find that it gives a degree of pleasure. Someone who takes pleasure in something likes it. It might be objected that pleasure explains liking in a way that liking does not explain pleasure. Does this not drive a wedge between the concept of pleasure and that of liking? It seems intelligible to say that we liked something because it gave pleasure. Is it not strange, however, to say that something gave pleasure because we liked it? S. Zink makes a similar point when he says[1]:

It would be intelligible, even if it were tautological, to say, 'I like the experience of malice because it gives me pleasure'; while it

---

[1] *The Concepts of Ethics*, p. 91.

would not be intelligible to say, 'I get pleasure from the experience of malice because I like it'.

To give the pleasure we get from something as the reason for our liking it is to put a stop to any further questioning. This is not because our liking has been explained, but because we have refused to go into the matter any further. To say 'it gives me pleasure; that's why I like it' is in the same category as an answer as 'I just like it, that's all'. There is the implication that we like it for its own sake and not as a means to an end, but we have not materially increased our questioner's knowledge of the reasons for our reaction. Zink is right in suggesting that 'I like the experience of malice because it gives me pleasure' is a tautology despite the appearance it has of telling us more of the situation. At first glance it looks very like an assertion such as 'I dislike having a tooth filled, because it gives me pain'. However, the fact that we get a sensation of pain does give an explanation for our dislike, whereas there seems to be no separate ingredient, called 'pleasure', which is added to the situation, over and above our liking it.

What of 'getting pleasure from x because we like x'? Is this intelligible? Someone might say that he gets pleasure from swimming, or, if he was talking of a particular episode, that he got pleasure from his swim, because he liked the swim. This must be distinguished from getting pleasure from a particular swim because of a liking for swimming in general, which would not be a tautology but a genuine explanation of sorts. It is also different from getting pleasure from the fact that we liked the swim (because, perhaps, we are pleased at our toughness). Although there can be episodes of liking, it is perhaps more usual to talk of *enjoying* a particular episode than of merely liking it. Nevertheless, anyone who attempts to give his liking for something on a single occasion as the reason for his pleasure does not seem to be saying anything unintelligible. He is certainly uninformative and even misleading in saying something which masquerades as an explanation. If he got pleasure from his swim, then of course he liked it, just as, if he liked it, he got some pleasure from it. His statement is as much a tautology when he explains his pleasure with his liking as the other way round. He might just as well be saying that he got pleasure from his swim because he got pleasure from his swim.

We have referred to *merely* liking an episode, and this does betray one of the usual reasons for any incongruity which arises when 'pleasure' and 'liking' are juxtaposed. If we like a sensation, we do not normally obtain great pleasure from it, just as, if we merely dislike a pain, we are not necessarily distressed by it. To say that we like something is often to put our experience at one end of the scale of pleasure. It is to say that we find the thing pleasant and nothing more. Getting pleasure from something, or finding the thing pleasureable is usually more than just liking it. I may like everything from which I get a lot of pleasure, but I do not get a great deal of pleasure from everything which I like. It is not a contradiction for someone to say: 'I like it, but I don't get a lot of pleasure from it.' It is a contradiction, if anyone who is not thinking of different aspects of the situation, says: 'I get some pleasure from it, but I don't like it.'

If all physical pleasures are sensations of different sorts which we like, it is clear that the concept of pleasure is completely dissimilar to that of pain. The kind of sensation in which we take pleasure is irrelevant to the concept. We cannot say that someone just 'feels pleasure', as someone can just 'feel pain'. No one can just 'be pleased', any more than they can just 'like'. We can, of course, merely say 'He is feeling pleased today', but there must be an answer to the very natural question 'What is he pleased about?' To say that he is not pleased about anything, but that he is just feeling pleased, would be odd, although the speaker might mean that the man is not pleased about anything in particular. He has a rosy attitude to life in general, instead of concentrating on one particular thing. He is in a good mood.

There are subtle differences between the various idioms with which we apparently talk about our pleasure. We can, for instance, be pleased at, with, by or about something. I can be pleased *about* somebody else's success, but I would be more likely to be pleased *with* my own. What I am pleased *about* is usually fairly remote from me whereas I can only be pleased *with* something for which I have some responsibility. All these are different from enjoyment. I might enjoy an activity like swimming or a sensation of some sort. We are not pleased at swimming, or if we are, we mean that we are pleased at the fact that we are swimming. This is distinct from taking pleasure in the activity of swimming—enjoying it or merely finding it pleasant. This suggests that each situation where we talk of 'enjoyment', 'pleasure', or 'being pleased', cannot necessarily be treated in the same way. If I say that I am pleased at something, I may mean that I approve of it, and I can certainly disapprove of things which I enjoy, and approve of things which I never find pleasant at all. We must be wary of assuming that every reference to 'being pleased' has anything directly to do with pleasure, just as it is wrong to assume that every reference to an episode of liking is linked with the concept of pleasure.

3. *Hedonic Tone*

Pleasure is not the name of a sensation. Can we, nevertheless, conclude that in each experience of taking pleasure in something, as opposed to merely approving of it in some way, there is the same ingredient which makes us say that the experience is one of *pleasure* and not something else? In that case, although our pleasure would have an 'object', the 'object' would be completely irrelevant to our decision as to whether we felt pleasure. What would count would be the presence or absence of the ingredient common to all experiences of pleasure. We have already agreed that such an ingredient could not be a sensation. It could not be a locatable feeling with a special quality. This view has, however, been refined in a way which was intended to keep pleasure and pain parallel.

In *Five Types of Ethical Theory* C. D. Broad puts forward a theory[1] which is reminiscent of the 'aspect theory' mentioned in Chapter I. He says that there is a quality which may be called 'hedonic tone', and which has 'the two determinate forms of Pleasantness and Unpleasantness'. He says:

'A pleasure' then is simply any mental event which has the pleasant form of hedonic tone, and 'a pain' is simply any kind of mental event which has the unpleasant form of hedonic tone.

We agreed that, apart from other considerations, this approach provides an inadequate analysis of physical pain, since not all unpleasant sensations are called pains. This objection does not apply to pleasure. We have seen that there is no important

[1] pp. 229–30.

distinction between physical pleasures and pleasant sensations. Was the mistake of holders of the aspect theory simply that in their eagerness to keep the two concepts parallel they assimilated pain to pleasure? Is the view of pleasure as an 'aspect' or 'tone' of an experience the correct one?

The theory entails that every experience which we call a pleasure would possess the same 'hedonic quality', although it would have other qualities as well. In so far as they are 'pleasures', various experiences have the same quality, although in other respects they are very different. Broad says: 'Hope, which is expectation of certain events, having a certain emotional tone, is plainly as much a pleasure as the sensation of smell which we get from a rose or violet.' In other words, according to Broad, both sensations and emotions can be pleasures, and they are pleasures for the same reason, namely that they both possess the same quality. He does not say what he means by quality, but he must at least be indicating that the experiences are similar enough in an important respect to be given the same description. It is, however, a great mistake to treat pleasantness (or unpleasantness) as a property. A closer examination of Broad's theory will illustrate this.

Although he mentions[1] the possibility of there being several 'determinate forms of pleasantness', he says[2]:

It is perfectly plain that there are 'differences of quality' among pleasures and pains in the sense that two experiences which were alike in hedonic quality might differ in non-hedonic quality (as a headache and a toothache do).

He thinks that pleasure can be the same whatever the experience it 'tones' or 'qualifies'. This is like the view which has been expressed[3] in a more recent analysis of the concept of pleasure. The writer says that pleasure is a quality, and continues:

One characteristic of pleasure is that it is always the same. . . . However the cause of it or the occasion for it may differ. . . . A man may experience pleasure at the sound of music or in the act of eating candy; one form of pleasure may persist longer, the other seem more intense; but pleasure is pleasure in every instance.

---

[1] *Five types of Ethical Theory*, p. 232.   [2] op. cit. p. 231.
[3] J. S. Feibleman in *The Role of Pleasure in Behavior*, ed. R. G. Heath, p. 252.

How plausible is this view? Even if episodes of pleasure are not accompanied by a special type of sensation, do they all possess the same 'quality' or 'tone'? The quality would be part of an experience and would be felt. Feibleman makes it quite clear that by a quality he means 'that property which is contained in a feeling'. When we feel this particular quality, we are feeling pleasure. The theory holds that the quality cannot be felt independently of another experience, and this does ensure that, although our pleasure is identified by the quality, it is always pleasure *in* something. Just as we cannot feel a quality which is not a quality of something, we cannot just feel pleasure. However, the experience of which the pleasure is supposed to be a quality cannot always be regarded as the 'object'. If I am overjoyed at some good news, it is not the hearing of the news, but the news itself, which I take pleasure in. I could not enjoy the experience of hearing the same news, if I knew the news was false. The theory does, however, circumvent Aristotle's objection[1] to pleasure being always the same. He maintained that if this were so, a pleasure from another source would help rather than hinder someone in an activity. The person eating candy with pleasure while listening to music would thereby enjoy the music more, instead of being distracted as seems to happen. If, however, pleasure is a quality, it clearly cannot be detached from a particular experience. It is not necessarily transferable between experiences.

The theory seems to have the unwelcome result that it is logically possible to feel the quality and not to be enjoying anything or taking pleasure in anything, even though we must be experiencing something else. Just as we know that we are feeling pain, without having to pay any attention to anything besides the sensation, it looks as if, on this theory, we can know we are feeling pleasure without paying any regard to anything besides the quality of our experience. If we feel it when we are listening to music, we are feeling pleasure (and presumably 'enjoying' the music), whatever we may think of the music. We may desperately want the music to stop, but that is irrelevant to whether we are feeling the distinctive quality of pleasure. If this is so, it must also be logically possible not to feel it when

---

[1] Nicomachean Ethics. 1175a, 21 ff.

we are showing every usual sign of pleasure in a situation where we think something is good in some respects and want it to continue. In that situation, according to the theory, I would have to conclude that I wasn't enjoying anything, because my experience was not tinged with the quality of pleasure. It is not altogether clear whether we are to regard the quality as the source of our pleasure. It seems from Broad's reference to 'pleasantness' as being one of the forms of hedonic tone as if it is being implied that the quality is what gives us pleasure. Broad talks of sensations which are 'pleasantly toned', and this just looks like another way of saying that we find them pleasant or like them. If Broad is saying that we like them because of the quality, he would have to concede that it would be logically possible for us to have the quality and not like it. If he wishes to insist that it is analytic that the quality is pleasant, and that it is present in every episode of pleasure, it is obvious that talk of the quality is just an alternative way of saying that we are taking pleasure in something.

Unless the quality is itself pleasant, it is difficult to see why it should be connected with pleasure. We may come to recognize it as the kind of feeling we have when we are enjoying something, just as 'throbs of fear' are sensations which we often have when afraid. We must, however, know what fear is before we can say that the throbs are throbs *of fear*, and not just throbs, and the same reasoning can be applied to the concept of hedonic tone. Unless we already know what it is to enjoy something, or take pleasure in it, how can we know that a particular quality is what Broad calls 'the pleasant form of hedonic tone'? If we do already know, this would suggest that an analysis of enjoyment in terms of hedonic tone is inadequate. Enjoyment would be something over and above feeling any particular quality. The quality would at best be an accompaniment of enjoyment; it could not itself be the enjoyment.

Broad is in fact making the same mistake with pleasure as he is with emotions in general. He thinks that we recognize from a specific quality in our experience when, for instance, we are afraid, and it is natural for him to hold the same view with regard to pleasure and pain. Indeed it seems a plausible view of pleasure, precisely because it results in pleasure and pain being coupled together in a neat fashion. The concept of the

hedonic tone enables Broad to say[1]: 'Headaches and tooth-
aches are both pains, for they both have unpleasant hedonic
tone.' It gives a reason why we group different types of sensations together as pains. The important thing, however, is
that they are *pains*, and not that they are unpleasant. Broad's
concentration on their unpleasantness instead of what we have
termed their 'pain-quality' leads him into trouble. He does not
see that the unpleasantness of a sensation is simply our dislike of
it. It is not a particular quality of the sensation any more than
the unpleasantness (or pleasantness) of any other experience is a
quality of the experience. Broad, however, treats the unpleasantness of all pain (mental and physical) as if it were the quality of
a sensation, and treats pleasure in the same way.

Just as the search for sensations with pleasure-quality proved
vain, it looks as if any search for a common felt ingredient in
experience of pleasure is misconceived. It was no accident that
Broad analysed pleasure in much the same way as he had
analysed emotions. We have seen that there is an emotional
component in most experiences of physical pain, and that mental
pain is itself an emotion. The concept of pleasure is not parallel
with that of physical pain. Is mental pain similar to pleasure in
any way? How far is pleasure an emotion? Like the emotions
pleasure takes an 'object'. It is clear that the way we regard the
'object' of our pleasure is of importance. To take pleasure in
something is to like it, and we cannot like something and at the
same time want to be rid of it for its own sake (although we may
have other reasons for objecting to it). We must think it good in
at least one respect, just as we must think the 'object' of our
distress to be bad in some way. We would not enjoy anything
which we completely disliked and thought wholly bad, and we
could not logically become distressed at something which we
thought good in every way. In this respect, at least, pleasure is
very like the emotions.

Emotions involve an element of disturbance. Mental pain,
such as distress, very obviously normally involves agitation.
We would scarcely believe anyone who said that they were
distressed and yet had no difficulty in remaining completely
calm. The concept of pleasure is not so amenable to generaliza-
tion. Someone who is 'filled with joy' is experiencing emotion

[1] *Five Types of Ethical Theory*, p. 230.

and yet he is clearly taking pleasure in something. Ecstasy is a state of extreme pleasure, and is hardly an instance of calmness. Enjoyment on the other hand need involve no element of disturbance. We would not expect someone who was enjoying gardening to be in transports of joy. He would normally be calm and collected, and could hardly be said to be in an emotional state. Some types of pleasure are more emotional than others. Ecstasy is at one end of the scale. At the other would be the kind of 'pleasure at' something, which suggested an approval of it, which was based on a considered judgement.

Like the emotions, pleasure does often involve feelings. There are thrills of pleasure, just as there are thrills of fear. As we have seen, however, the feelings are neither the 'object' nor the defining feature of our pleasure. In this respect, as in others, pleasure should be likened to *mental* pain. We must resist the ever-present temptation to conclude, from the fact that pleasure and pain are often coupled, that there must be sensations of pleasure, on the model of sensations of pain. We must also resist the opposite temptation, to which the aspect theorists succumbed. We must not assume that because there are no sensations of pleasure, there are no sensations of pain.

VII

PREFRONTAL LEUCOTOMY

1. *The Effects of Leucotomy*

W E must now resume our discussion of striking cases of abnormal reactions to noxious stimuli. It is often far from clear whether the patients are feeling any pain, or if they are, whether they dislike it. In recent years, the operation of prefrontal leucotomy (or lobotomy) has apparently given clear evidence of the sensation of pain being felt without any emotional accompaniments. The purpose of the operation is to cut the nerve fibres which connect the front of the brain with the rest. This has been found to have far-reaching effects on the personality, and for this reason surgeons are nowadays reluctant to perform it. It has often in the past been used to relieve intractable pain in fatal diseases (quite often when a patient has become addicted to 'pain-killing' drugs). It has usually been said that after the operation the patients claim to have pain but show no disposition to manifest 'pain-behaviour.' As Baier states[1]: 'In cases of prefrontal lobotomy, patients claim that they have the same feelings as before, but they no longer mind.' Similarly Armstrong refers to such cases and says[2]: 'There are situations where people report that they have pains but they say that the pain is not giving them any sort of concern.' This is the 'official story' that many philosophers have accepted and tried to fit into their theories about the concept of pain. There have however been others who have claimed that, as the operation makes people 'simple-minded', we need take no notice of anything the patients say.

In this chapter the case-histories of prefrontal leucotomy will be examined to see if the 'official story' can be accepted (or if, at the other extreme, patients are so demented that nothing they say can be taken seriously). In our previous terminology,

---

[1] 'Pains', *Australasian Journal of Philosophy*, 40 (1962), 7.
[2] *Bodily Sensations*, p. 101.

the 'official story' says that the patients recognize their sensation as being one with pain-quality but do not dislike it, and
are not in any way distressed at it. We have already accepted
that this is a logical possibility, and have suggested that a case
of asymbolia for pain, as reported, does provide us with a
concrete example of such a situation. Does prefrontal leucotomy provide us with more instances? In fact this is a more
difficult question to answer than the 'official story' might
indicate. The operation does not have uniform effects. Indeed
sometimes it is a complete failure, and does not relieve suffering
at all. Even in individual cases, there is often conflicting
evidence—not just as to whether the patient is feeling pain at
all, but also whether he is disliking it or not, and whether it is as
he claims.

An example of a post-leucotomy case at its most puzzling is
reported by Robinson and Freeman.[1] They say of one patient:

She told the psychologist she was not having any pain in her face:
but when the surgeon came in and enquired, she insisted it was bad,
though she looked relaxed and peaceful. In order to display her
contrasting reaction to unexpected pain, he suddenly pulled off a
piece of the adhesive tape that held her bandage to her head. She
let out a lusty yell.

Our first problem is whether she was in pain or not. If she
looked relaxed and peaceful, we can assume that, if she did
feel pain, she did not dislike it very much. What are we to make
of her claims, first to be without pain, and then to have 'bad'
pain? Her statement that she was not having any pain suggests
that she was not just talking of that moment but of her general
condition, and presumably her answer to the surgeon was
intended to be about that too. We are thus faced with a straight
contradiction. She both claimed that she was in a state of pain
and that she was not. Her reference to 'bad' pain suggests
that she meant she was distressed at it, and yet this was contradicted by her appearance, which was certainly not of someone who was making a desperate effort to restrain any signs of
distress. Finally, her reaction to sudden ordinary pain was
normal, or, if anything, less inhibited than normal. It is clear
that the removal of the adhesive caused her pain, which she

[1] *Psychosurgery and the Self*, p. 71.

disliked very much, and this was expressed in her yell. Her case is thus distinct from that of the man with asymbolia for pain, who apparently did not dislike *any* pain. In this, at least, leucotomy patients show a fairly standard reaction. The operation may affect the pain of their disease in varying ways, but it does not appear to stop them feeling and disliking other pains which may occur for a moment. Indeed such patients are often less inhibited than is usual in expressing their dislike or distress. This very fact may make it more difficult to dismiss, on the grounds that they do not understand the concept, whatever they may say about the pain they claim to feel and not dislike. If in one situation they exhibit normal 'pain-behaviour' (in response to a normal cause of pain) when they talk of pain, why should we refuse to accept their claims to feel pain, which does not carry with it even an inclination to the normal behavioural accompaniments? Abnormal situations need not be unintelligible ones. If it was just a question of using the word 'pain' normally before the operation and abnormally after it, we might well suspect that the individual's conceptual memory had been adversely affected. The fact that in many instances the concept is applied normally after the operation would seem to rule out this escape route.

Perhaps all this is answered by saying quite simply that the operation has made the patients simple-minded. Because they use the word normally one moment, one must not expect that they will be at all consistent the next. Someone who claims to be in a state of pain, and almost immediately denies that she is, and who claims to have 'bad' pain, and yet looks relaxed, is so muddled that a 'proper' use of the word need not rule out the possibility of an immediate misuse. This may be true of the case just quoted, and of some others, but it is definitely not true of the majority. Whatever untoward psychological effects the operation has, many patients after it remain reasonably lucid and consistent. When this is not so, surgeons do not hesitate to say so. For instance one group[1] tell of a man who 'reported on questioning that he had pain in his leg. This was said in an expressionless manner. A week later the patient stated he had no pain, not even in his legs.' It is true that the pain may have

[1] Koskoff, Dennis, Lazovick and Wheeler in *Res. Publ. Ass. nerv. ment. Dis.* 27 (1948), 729.

stopped during the week, but it is hardly likely with a permanent disease. We might therefore suspect that the man is too muddled to be consistent, and in fact on general grounds the authors concluded that there was a 'postoperative intellectual defect', aggravated by severe meningitis.

It is significant that this patient mentioned pain only after questioning. A very definite pattern emerges in leucotomy cases over the patients' readiness to complain of pain. Before the operation it is common for them to find grave difficulty in paying attention to anything but the pain, and this is reflected in their conversation. The case already quoted from Robinson and Freeman is an example of this. Before the operation, we are told, the patient[1] 'described herself as nearly frantic with the pain. . . . She talked at great length about her symptoms. She continually interrupted herself to talk about her pain. She had her handbag full of medications.' After the operation, her obsession ceased, and indeed a general apathy set in, epitomized by her remarks: 'I never think about the past and I don't care about the future.'[2] Most patients appear to pay so little attention to their pain (if they have any) after the operation, that only a direct question which forces them to focus their attention brings out any reference to it. Robinson and Freeman say[3]: 'Most of these patients postoperatively will report pain when questioned but, unquestioned, are uncomplaining and no longer demand narcotics. Apparently the sensations of pain remain, but the dread of it is gone.' Has dislike of it also vanished? Might it remain as the patients' concern is narrowed to the immediate present, while fear of the pain and its significance vanishes? We shall consider this possibility, but first we must ask how far the operation affects the actual intensity of the pain, as any change would probably also affect their dislike (if any).

We have previously suggested that the intensity of sensations should be analysed in terms of the attention we are forced to pay to them. If this is right, the operation of leucotomy appears to cut the intensity of the permanent pain of the patients (though not of accidental pains). Before the operation they appear completely unable to pay any sustained attention to

[1] *Psychosurgery and the Self*, p. 70.
[2] op. cit. p. 72.
[3] op. cit. p. 68.

anything else. After the operation, they appear to have great difficulty in paying attention to the pain. What do the patients themselves say or imply about the sensation's intensity? It is reported of one woman[1]:

> She was confused but looked content and complained little. When questioned she usually said the arm 'pained', but did not volunteer the information. When she was questioned further about the pain she stated that the pain was present but that she gave it less attention and it did not concern her.

Here again, it is possible to seize on the word 'confused', and to dismiss the whole report as being merely about the muddled meanderings of a near-imbecile. This seems rather cavalier as she seems perfectly consistent in what she says, and her appearance is in accord with her words. She certainly claims to feel pain, but her apparent contentment supports her claim that it does not 'concern' her. How far the claim that her arm 'pained' suggests that she found it unpleasant and disliked it is hard to ascertain. Probably neither she nor the physiologists reporting the case made a distinction between the two uses of 'pain'. Certainly a lack of 'concern' may mean a lack of worry rather than a lack of all dislike, although here her lack of 'pain-behaviour' may suggest the latter. For our immediate purposes, her claim to give the pain 'less attention' is the most interesting. This could well indicate a decrease of intensity in the sensation. There is, however, another interpretation.

2. *Leucotomy and Anxiety*

In our previous discussion of the relation of intensity and attention it was admitted that intensity could not be tied conceptually to the amount of attention we actually *do* pay. We could pay a great deal of attention to a pain, the significance of which was a source of worry to us. It was claimed that it was the ease or difficulty with which we would be distracted from the sensation which provided the link with intensity. A possible objection to this would be that it might be very difficult to forget one sensation (which might *demand* our attention) while we could comparatively easily be distracted from another sensation, and the reason for this would not be a difference in

---

[1] Wolff and Hardy, *Physiological Reviews*, 27 (1947), 193.

intensity but in our fear (perhaps even our terror) of the meaning of the first pain. If we saw that our fears were mistaken, the sensation need not necessarily change, and our new-found ease in disregarding it would show that it was not as intense as the second sensation. In this case, therefore, the actual difficulty we had in trying not to pay attention to the sensation is irrelevant. What is relevant is the difficulty (or ease) we would have, if our beliefs about the significance of the sensation changed and the sensation did not. It might be that leucotomy strips away the beliefs about the meaning of the pain (its threat of an early death, for instance) and narrows the patients' view to such an extent that they pay attention to the sensation in proportion to its intensity and not to their fears about it.

Do case-histories bear this out? If it is correct, we might expect patients to pay less attention to the pain after the operation, and yet to claim that the intensity of the pain was as it was before the operation. The implication of this is, of course, that their pains were not of excruciating intensity before the operation despite appearances. Their emotional state was directed as much at the significance of the pain as at the pain itself. Anxiety could be supposed to have played at least as large a part as distress. As usual, no consistent story can be culled from the accounts of what patients say. There is evidence, however, which suggests that in many cases anxiety is relieved, while the sensation (quality, intensity and all, presumably) remains the same. Freeman and Watts[1] say of one woman:

When she was asked about the pain shortly after the operation she replied: 'Sure, It's exactly like it was before.' 'But you don't complain any more,' we suggested. 'What's the use,' she answered, 'I can't do anything about it, so it doesn't do any good to complain.'

In other words someone whose thoughts were dominated by her pain before the operation could accept it after the operation in an apathetic manner. Her attention was not demanded by it in the same way, and yet she claimed that the sensation was 'exactly like it was before'. Another case reported by the authors shows clearly how fear of pain can become more intolerable than the pain itself. The patient said: 'I guess I could stand the pains if it wasn't for the thought of them coming on.' After leucotomy,

[1] *Lancet*, i (1946), 955.

'he continued to have attacks, but described them as twinges and never complained about them'. He must have disliked them, however, as he did take aspirin for them. The use of the word 'twinge' suggests that the pain (as they were presumably twinges of pain) was not very intense and that each attack was short-lived. It is an interesting speculation whether he might have described the sensations as twinges before the operation, if it had not been for his general state of anxiety. His admission that he could stand the pains if it was not for his fear of them suggests that they were not of great intensity, and that 'twinge' might not have been an inappropriate word to apply.

Elsewhere[1] the same authors report another case where, a year after the operation, 'The patient stated that the pain was just as it was before the operation. And yet she does not talk about it, she is rather carefree, and her arm is a nuisance, rather than a constant reminder of her permanent invalidism.' Once again, we have a patient's claim that the pain was unchanged (and this must refer both to its quality and intensity). Nevertheless the demand on her attention has gone, and the pain can be disregarded by her. If we accept that the intensity is unchanged, this must mean that her condition before the operation was primarily one of anxiety (and with an atrophic arm she had good reason for this).

Other cases show how all anxiety about the future, and hence about the significance of the pain, disappears after the operation. In their book on *Psychosurgery* Freeman and Watts quote an instance of this.[2] The patient followed a normal pattern of leucotomy and did not complain or ask for hypodermics after the operation. He did admit he had pain when specifically asked about it. 'When asked if he knew he was going to die', we are told, 'he replied, "Sure everybody has to die, don't they?" His calm acceptance of pain and impending death continued until he died three months later.' Similarly J. C. Nemiah[3] tells of a patient who was 'constantly depressed and anxious' before the operation. 'This was manifested', we are told, 'in his facial expression, in the loudness and emphasis of his voice, as well as in the anger and crying which he exhibited when he talked about his pain, and when he momentarily touched on his concern

[1] Watts and Freeman, *Res. Publ. Ass. nerv. ment. Dis.* 27 (1948), 717.
[2] *Psychosurgery*, p. 360.   [3] *Psychosomatic Medicine*, 24 (1962), 75–80.

about his paraplegia.' There was a considerable change after
the operation. 'When speaking of either his pain or disability
his voice was flat and lifeless, and he showed no evidence of
anxiety or depression.'

This patient had plenty to be anxious about. He was going to
be paralysed for the rest of his life, and would find it physically
impossible to go back to his old job. His old life had completely
disintegrated, and he would have to start afresh. His pain became the focus of his worries before leucotomy. It was the
'object', though not the cause, of much of his emotion, and it
became clear that the patient irrationally thought that if only
it would disappear all would be well. Nemiah reports what
happened when anyone tried to get the patient to talk about
his paralysis and its implications. 'He would appear distressed,
anxious and tearful. However, he would vigorously deny that
these were problems for him, that he had thought about them,
or that he was in any way concerned. Instead he would usually
respond with a highly emotional complaint about the pains
in his legs.' His self-deception is made all the more obvious by
the fact that his complaints of pain started suddenly, 'when a
few days after his embarking on a programme of rehabilitation,
the patient had been badly confronted with the fact that his
paralysis was permanent.' It is clear that he refused to admit
even to himself that he was anxious about his predicament,
and directed his concern at the pain itself, the quality and intensity of which did not presumably warrant such an emotional
state. That he was really anxious about his paralysis is shown by
his demeanour when asked about it.

If it affected anxiety, leucotomy could be expected to have a
considerable impact on this patient, as it did. The pain itself
need not have been diminished at all for his distress at it to be
lessened, if the distress was indeed largely the product of the
anxiety he refused to admit. The operation helped him to face
his disability and the consequences, and yet not react emotionally when he thought of them. Because of this, Nemiah claims:
'There was no further need of pain as a substitute for his concern
over his life situation, and as a carrier of the emotions resulting
from this concern. As a consequence, the intensity of the pains
and the vehemence of his complaints about them was markedly
diminished.' If his distress at the pains had been lessened, we

would expect the vehemence of his complaints to follow suit. They were, after all, an expression of his distress. What is more dubious is Nemiah's assumption that the intensity of the pains had been diminished. If, as we have seen, the patient's distress had causes other than the intensity or quality of the sensation, there is no reason to suppose that the decrease in his distress after the removal of these causes was in any way because the 'object' had changed. His lack of distress after the operation would be merely an indication of how disproportionate to the pains his distress had been before leucotomy. However, there is the complication of the apparent effect which leucotomy has even on the dislike of the sensation for its own sake.

The patient in Nemiah's case still said his legs hurt after the operation, and did not claim that his pains were any better. This is in accord with a familiar pattern in post-leucotomy patients. The leucotomy diminishes their anxiety, but does not lessen their pain. This is usually so marked that one group of investigators[1] recommend leucotomy only in cases of an 'excessive psychological reaction of the anxious, depressive or ruminative type'. They say: 'The more likely it is that the patient is suffering from severe physical pain, the less likely it is that leucotomy will help him.' This is all neat and consistent, but unfortunately there are patients who claim that their pain is less severe after the operation, and the ease with which they can pay attention to other things might seem to support them. Falconer says of one patient[2]: 'He made no spontaneous mention of his pain. But when questioned he would confess that he still felt pain in his right leg, although usually it was not now severe.' Falconer enlarges on this by reporting: 'Usually he says this pain is slight and of no moment, but occasionally he says that it is severe.' As the patient never made any spontaneous mention of his pain, it is hard to imagine that he was in severe pain at all. If he could easily disregard it, it was not severe, so that at least part of what he said about his pain is questionable. Falconer comments: 'The observation that his pain now seems of diminished intensity probably derives from the fact that formerly he was preoccupied with his pain,

[1] Elithorn, Glithero and Slater, *Journal of Neurology, Neorosurgery and Psychiatry*, 21 (N.S. 1958), 249–61.
[2] Falconer, *Res. Publ. Ass. nerv. ment. Dis.* 27 (1948), 712.

and consequently regarded and described it in superlatives.'
If however he had his attention drawn to the pain, as opposed
to its significance (and he 'regarded and described' it as intense), then the pain *was* intense, and no one else can say that
it was not. We may well have to accept in this case that the
intensity of the pain did diminish. We have observed before
that leucotomy does not have uniform effects, and some patients
deny pain completely after it. It is quite reasonable to suppose
that in some cases (which are probably untypical) the pain
itself becomes less intense.

3. *Leucotomy and Dislike of Pain*

If anxiety is usually eradicated, is dislike of the sensation in
itself affected? Obviously, if the pain is less strong, a patient
will dislike it less. What if it remains at the same intensity?
Once again, there is conflicting evidence. It seems fairly usual
for patients no longer to demand narcotics, and this might
suggest that even if their pain is still present, they do not want
to be rid of it. If someone knows how he could stop something
and makes no effort to do so, it would generally appear that he
does not want to. As we have seen, someone who does not want
to be rid of his pain could hardly be said to dislike it. The
tendency of patients to report pain after leucotomy, in a matter-
of-fact tone of voice also suggests that they have no dislike of it
but have a completely neutral attitude towards it.

Physiologists never appear to ask whether the patient dislikes
the pain he says he feels. Presumably they think it would be a
silly question. For example, Elithorn, Glithero and Slater[1],
after a few words on the importance of leucotomy in relieving
anxiety, say: 'The typical post-leucotomy syndrome in cases of
intractable pain is one in which the patient still makes complaints of severe pain, but shows at the same time an affect
inappropriately cheerful.' This is strictly speaking a contradiction. If someone 'complains' of severe pain, their 'affect' is
hardly cheerful. The investigators seem to be assuming that
any mention of pain must be a 'complaint', and indeed this is
a confusion often made. It means that it is very difficult when
someone is reported as 'complaining' of pain to decide whether
he is grumbling about it and wants to be rid of it, or is simply

[1] *Journal of Neurology, Neurosurgery and Psychiatry*, 21 (N.S. 1958), 249 ff.

saying, 'I have a pain.' One report[1], for example, says of a patient: 'He is considerably better than he was prior to the operation, but occasionally he complains of pain momentarily and soon forgets about it. He does not require any medication.' His lack of desire for drugs to relieve the pain might suggest he does not dislike it, while the use of the word 'complain' makes us wonder if perhaps there are not moments when he does become distressed at it.

There are cases reported where the dissociation of pain from 'reaction' is far from complete, and they could suggest that although anxiety has been removed dislike has not. One case-history says[2]: 'Although he never spontaneously mentions his pain, whenever he is asked about it directly, he replies each time that his pain is "terrible" or "unbearable". Yet next moment he will seem to have forgotten it.' His use of these words suggests that he is greatly distressed at the pain. It certainly would not appear that he had a neutral attitude towards it. 'My pain is unbearable but I don't dislike it', is a contradiction. Yet apart from his use of the words, there was nothing to suggest he was in any agony. Falconer comments: 'He seems oblivious of the fact that his operation has changed him from an extremely miserable man into one whose appearances and reactions suggest content-ment. A chance acquaintance would regard him as a normal elderly man without obvious peculiarities and mannerisms.' Even the fact that he never talked of his pain spontaneously would suggest that it was far from unbearable. He was presum-ably talking of a continuing pain and not of momentary attacks. To say of such a pain that it is 'unbearable' and then to appear to have forgotten about it is puzzling. It seems hardly possible by any criterion that he was suffering 'terrible' or 'unbearable' pain. It is important that he is extremely untypical of leucotomy patients in his use of these epithets, while showing no other signs of distress.

Other cases show different types of inconsistency. Wolff[3] describes some patients after the operation: 'When asked they say, yes, they had quite severe pain, and yet they made no spontaneous complaints, and required no analgesics for relief

---

[1] Bonner, Cobb, Sweet and White, *Psychosomatic Medicine*, 14 (1952), 395.
[2] Falconer, *Res. Publ. Ass. nerv. ment. Dis.* 27 (1948), 709.
[3] *Res. Publ. Ass. nerv. ment, Dis.*, 27 (1948), 764.

as they lay quietly in bed.' This so far follows the typical pattern. The patients have to be asked, before they admit to pain. This would indicate that it is not absorbing their attention and is therefore not very severe. We might wonder whether their description of it as 'quite severe' might not be putting the intensity a bit high. The fact that they require no analgesics suggests that they do not want to be rid of the pain, and their lack of dislike or distress is further emphasized by their quietness in bed. However Wolff goes on to say: 'Often they disturbed the ward by their agonizing shrieks when they were turned over in bed. A moment or so later they were seemingly comfortable again. When asked about the pain they said it was of no importance.' The 'agonizing shrieks' were no doubt partly the result of the general lack of inhibition which is a feature of the post-leucotomy state. This would probably mean that they would appear to be in a more distressed condition than they really were, because they would make no effort to restrain any inclination to cry out. The shrieks do, however, indicate a dislike of the pain at that moment, which does not appear to be usually present. Presumably they were given considerably more pain for a moment when they were turned over. Normal patients with an organic disease would find the same.

Why should the leucotomy patients dislike the momentary pain, and yet be indifferent to the pain of their disease? It could be claimed that the patients were not in continuous pain, and that they just had momentary recurrences when they were moved. This theory, however, involves dismissing their reports of pain which, we have maintained, are quite intelligible. On the other hand, the patients might have some continuous pain which was so slight as not to provoke much reaction. In that case, only when they are moved would their pain become sufficient to distress them. This is more plausible as the patients do not usually seem to have their attention drawn to the pain. The implication would be that leucotomy only influences the patients' anxiety, and not their dislike of pain, since the argument assumes that the only reason the patients do not dislike the continuous pain is that it is not strong enough. Is the report intelligible, on the other hand, if leucotomy does stop patients disliking the pain of their disease? It must be remembered that it does not in any way affect their immediate attitude to ordinary, momentary pain (as when they bang against something). On this interpretation, the patients behave as would be expected towards their continuous pain. They accept it in an apathetic way; it does not concern them, and they do not want to be rid of it. Only when they are turned over do they express dislike of pain, and this might be because of the sudden increase in the amount they feel. The pain is no longer regarded as the pain they accept (because of their leucotomy) as a part of their life; it is thought of as sudden accidental pain—to which leucotomy patients typically have an exaggerated reaction. Their subsequent assertion that this was of no importance indicates that the total emotional reaction of patients to the momentary attacks lasts only as long as the attack. They are incapable of any anxiety about it, and obviously do not associate the pain of being turned over with the permanent pain of their disease.

The inability to relate different features of their experience is the most pronounced effect of leucotomy on patients. It is this which makes their anxiety disappear, as they are unable to see the significance of the pain they feel. This shows itself in other ways besides the change in their attitude to their pain, and results in general irresponsibility and fecklessness. It is reported of one post-leucotomy case[1]: 'Shortly after discharge, he attempted to fill a fuel-tank with oil while smoking, and burned himself to death.' The operation had made him incapable of relating his smoking to the filling of the tank, although, presumably, before it he would have been well aware of the danger. The same group of physiologists also tell of a woman who was unable to see the significance of her symptoms: 'Fourteen months after her unilateral leucotomy, she almost died from pelvic peritonitis, the symptoms of which she had neglected for six days.' Both of these cases are very similar to one which is summed up as follows: 'Although she had all the facts in a given situation, nevertheless she was unable to relate them to each other in a meaningful way.' It can be seen that a patient's lack of anxiety about his pain is part of the general pattern. The pain is there but he cannot comprehend its implications. Freeman and Watts say[2]: 'Pain may be present, but when divorced

---

[1] Bonner, Cobb, Sweet and White, *Psychosomatic Medicine*, 14 (1952), 388.
[2] *Lancet*, i (1946), 955.

from its implications—insecurity, guilt, death—it then becomes bearable, and may be accepted with fortitude.'

This brings us back to the question whether post-leucotomy patients do dislike the pain of their disease. Do they need 'fortitude' to accept the pain, or is it just a neutral sensation for them, like a tingle, or a heart-beat—something they feel, without having any emotional attitude towards it? Is the relief of anxiety the whole story, or just a large part of it? The 'official story' we mentioned at the beginning of the chapter ignores this and merely holds that the main effect of leucotomy is to stop the patient disliking pain, so that he has feelings of pain which do not bother him in any way. Again and again, however, we have seen that anxiety and fear of the significance of the pain, rather than distress at the pain itself, have caused the greatest suffering before leucotomy and have been most noticeably relieved after it. Watts and Freeman say of patients after leucotomy[1]: 'Fear seemed to have gone. The pain was still present, but it was a sensation rather than a threat.' Instead of being the dominant factor in their lives, the pain often becomes a mere 'twinge' for which they take aspirin (a sign that they still do dislike it to some extent and want to be rid of it). It is clear, however, that the effects of leucotomy are far from uniform and, whilst relief of anxiety is the main purpose and result of the operation, sufficient apathy is often induced to make the patients bother as little about their permanent pain as about its significance, although any sudden change in the pain, or any new pain, is liable to evoke an immediate (and superficial) reaction. They see and care little for anything outside the actual present.

Leucotomy is not primarily intended to relieve distress at very severe pain. Elithorn, Glithero and Slater say[2]: 'In considering cases of intractable pain for leucotomy, it must be remembered that the pain will not be relieved and that normal people cannot by leucotomy be made inattentive to severe pain, unless the operation produces a very definite dementia.' It is unclear what being 'inattentive to severe pain' would be. It is possible to force one's attention to other matters and forget one's pain, or at least not to let it dominate one's attention, but the

---

[1] *Res. Publ. Ass. nerv. ment. Dis.* 27 (1948), 715.

[2] *Journal of Neurology, Neurosurgery and Psychiatry*, 21 (N.S. 1958), 249 ff.

authors are obviously not thinking of such strength of will. They are envisaging a situation where the pain remains severe, but where it is no longer so noticeable, and where the patients can easily turn their minds to other things. This must be a contradiction. The pain logically cannot be as severe any longer, if the analysis of the intensity of sensations in terms of their noticeability is correct. If leucotomy had any effect on severe pain, it would either have to reduce the intensity of the sensation, or relieve and perhaps completely remove the patient's distress at it, as well as his anxiety. The latter possibility is more in accord with the usual effects of the operation, and it might be what the authors have in mind. Someone who is no longer distressed by his pain might appear to be no longer as absorbed in it, although his attention might be drawn to it just as much. The authors have probably fallen into the popular trap of confusing the intensity of a pain with the strength of our dislike of it.

4. *Intensity and Dislike*

There is some difficulty in describing what it would be to have one's attention irresistibly drawn to a pain, and yet not to be distressed at it, or indeed to mind it in the slightest. This must be logically possible if it is contingent that pains are disliked, and if very intense pains are those pains which most demand our attention. It would to some extent be comparable with the very noticeable thumping of one's heart in a terrifying situation. We could not help noticing it, but the sensation itself need be neither pleasant nor unpleasant. There is, however, no analogy between intense pain and intense fear. Intense emotions are not like intense sensations, and when we experience them, our attention is not directed to particular feelings. They are rather instances of great disturbance and agitation in a particular setting, and our attention is given to the 'object'. I could not be absorbed with my feelings of fear and yet unconcerned about the 'object' of my fear, as I can be absorbed with a pain and yet not distressed at it. In fact, if I was unconcerned, I could not be afraid, and the feelings which may have drawn my attention could not be called feelings of *fear*. They might even be distracting me from the 'object' of my fear, and hence from my fear generally.

There are those who might admit that pain of moderate intensity could logically be a neutral, or even a pleasant, sensation. They would deny, however, that intense pain need not be disliked. It is always very unpleasant, they would maintain, and as a consequence of this someone in intense pain is always to be pitied. Certainly it is hard to over-emphasize the abnormality of someone who was not distressed at intense pain, and did not even dislike it, but an abnormality is not a conceptual impossibility. It is sometimes difficult to see whether those who take exception to the idea of intense pain not being disliked are in fact saying it is logically or only humanly impossible. Are they saying that it could not happen, or only that it does not happen? It is apparent that they are often not sure themselves. For example, the writer of one article[1] suggests that it is intelligible to ask masochists whether a certain pain was unpleasant. He continues: 'But the question could make sense, even when addressed to a masochist, only in respect of ostensibly locatable bodily pains below a certain degree of intensity. . . . We have another word altogether for those great degrees of pain which it is unlikely that the most enthusiastic masochist ever goes in for: the word "agony".' He claims that it is unintelligible to ask a masochist whether a pain above a certain degree of intensity was unpleasant. There could be no room for even logical doubt that it was, according to him. Yet two sentences later he is only suggesting that it is 'unlikely' that a masochist 'goes in for' very intense pains. In other words, it is improbable that it happens often. This is a marked shift, since what is unlikely can happen sometimes, in contrast with what is unintelligible. Unfortunately the issue is confused still further by his use of the word 'agony', which is one of the words that carries with it the notion of adverse emotional reaction, as well as of a sensation of pain. 'Agony', or an 'agonizing' pain, certainly suggests that the sensation is an intense one, but in addition their use entails that the intense sensation is positively distressing. It may therefore be logically possible for a masochist to find a very high degree of pain pleasant. (We shall discuss in the next chapter whether this is in fact a correct description of what happens in masochism.) It is not logically possible for him to find 'agony' pleasant, as the application of the word

[1] R. J. O'Shaughnessy, 'Enjoying and Suffering', *Analysis*, vol 26 (April 1966), 158.

'agony' to an intense pain has prejudged that particular issue. To deny that it is merely 'unlikely' that a masochist likes 'agony' is not to say anything about the logical properties of 'intense pain'. It is a result of the meaning of the word 'agony'. The fact that one can use it naturally in situations of mental pain (as when one is in an 'agony of despair', or is faced with an 'agonizing choice') indicates that the idea of distress predominates in it, over that of a sensation of pain. It is certainly possible for the word to be used in situations of distress, where there is no physical pain, but impossible where there is a sensation of pain, without any distress accompanying it.

Part of the difficulty in describing intense pain, which is not unpleasant in itself, lies in the fact that one ground we have for calling pain 'an evil' would still remain. Intense pain demands our attention, and hinders us from concentrating on other matters. Although distress and anxiety exacerbate this, their alleviation or complete removal does not solve the basic problem. We simply cannot give our full attention to two things at once. The more intense our pain is, the less able we are to concentrate on what we want. Loud noises perhaps offer a parallel. A loud noise does not necessarily have to be distressing or in any way unpleasant, but there is a logical link between the apparent loudness of a sudden noise and its demand on our attention. The louder it seems to sound to us, the more difficult it is to ignore it. Of course, if we are deaf, a loud noise will appear to be a quiet sound, and will not catch our attention very easily. If a noise does impinge on our attention and break our train of thought, we may very well be annoyed. Even then we may not dislike the noise, but only the fact that we are interrupted. Similarly, if I feel an intense pain, and do not dislike it in any way, I may still dislike its demand on my attention, and even be distressed at it. I might think it an evil, if it continued for long, because, unpleasant or not, it would still be a great and unnecessary distraction. The 'object' of my emotion, however, would not be the pain itself, nor any implications it may carry of disease or death. It would merely be the fact that I am distracted. If I did not mind being distracted, and had nothing else on hand to which I particularly wanted to pay attention, I would not dislike the experience in any way. However, for people who wanted to live a normal life, the removal of the emotional element in the experience of pain, without any diminution in the intensity of the sensation, would provide only a limited advantage. Frustration and annoyance at the continuing distraction could well replace distress at the sensation.

VIII

'NON-PAINFUL PAIN' AND 'PLEASANT PAIN'

1. *'Non-Painful Pain'*

WE do not usually dislike moderate pain as much as severe pain, and we are not so ready to take measures (such as limping) to alleviate something which does not concern us very much. This is a fact of normal experience, but it does raise the question whether our dislike of pain may not disappear before the pain does. Might we recognize that a sensation which is only just noticeable has pain-quality and yet is not unpleasant? The experiments of physiologists measuring the threshold of pain suggest that this does happen, although it is instructive to see how they get into conceptual difficulties if they do not clearly distinguish between pain-quality and the emotional reaction.

There is a general bewilderment amongst subjects and experiments about how to describe a sensation which is the same in every respect as what they would call a 'pain' except for the fact that they do not dislike it. This is implicit in one physiologist's description of the phenomenon[1]:

There can be differentiated at successive stages of intensity of stimulation . . . first a nondescript threshold contact sense, then prick, merging gradually into pain, which, under experimental conditions at least, is recognized as 'painful,' i.e. is perceived without emotional protest; followed finally by a degree of this same painful sensation which becomes a definitely objectionable experience, and induces an emotional reaction of protest and other physiological evidence of an avoidance or protective reaction.

The writer's uneasiness is betrayed by his use of 'painful' to describe a sensation with pain-quality, which is *not* unpleasant. Not content with his strained use of the word, on the next page of his article Bishop talks of 'non-painful "pain" ', meaning

---

[1] G. H. Bishop, *Physiological Reviews*, 26 (1946), 98.

pain which is not unpleasant. In the one instance he uses the word 'painful' to refer solely to the quality of the sensation, in the other he uses it to describe our reaction to the quality. Clearly he is also worried about denying that 'pain' is 'painful', even though he finds himself driven to it. He puts 'pain' inside inverted commas, as if to suggest that if it is not 'painful', it cannot really be 'pain'. He naturally feels that he may be asserting what is a straight contradiction, of the same type as 'non-coloured colour'. What the first part denies the second asserts. Certainly the phrase 'non-painful pain' is needlessly confusing, but it need not be regarded as self-contradictory, if it is realized that while the noun refers to the sensation the adjective refers to our reaction to it. If sensation and reaction are clearly differentiated we shall not be tempted to apply to the one a word which is more appropriate to the other.

Bishop's difficulties in his terminology arise from his reluctance to face and accept explicitly the possibility of a sensation which is not unpleasant being called pain without qualification. There is in his description of the results of experiments an unstated assumption that pain must logically be disliked. When the subjects' descriptions of their sensations challenge this, it is not surprising that some confusion develops. There is general agreement in reports of similar experiments that, whereas there is a definite change in the quality of the sensation as its intensity increases, it occurs before the sensation becomes unpleasant. Bishop himself says[1]: 'The division point is between touch and prick, not between touch and pain.' He reports that 'prick' merges gradually into 'pain' and that there is no recognizable change in the sensation once it has become a 'prick'. It just becomes more intense, and our attitude to it changes. Bishop distinguishes between 'prick' and 'pain', but it is apparent that his sole ground is his reluctance to use 'pain' for a sensation which is not unpleasant. For him 'prick' becomes 'pain' when the element of 'emotional protest' is introduced. This, however, suggests that pain is merely a pricking sensation which is disliked, whereas it is surely possible to claim to feel a pricking sensation, and to dislike it, while denying that it is actually a 'pain'. Bishop's use of the adjective 'painful' in connection with a 'prick' suggests that there is something about the sensation

[1] *Physiological Reviews*, 26 (1946), 88.

which tempts him to call it a pain. Only his conceptual pre-judices hold him back, and it is obvious that he is using the word 'prick' to describe sensations with pain-quality.

Other physiologists encounter the same phenomenon, when conducting similar experiments. With the same assumptions about the concept of pain as Bishop, they naturally encounter the same difficulty. C. A. Keele[1] reports on the sensations which occur when different amounts of chemical solutions are applied to an exposed blister base. He says that in his experience, although the sensation becomes unpleasant after being neutral or even pleasant, the quality of the sensation is 'continuous in most ways' right through. He concludes: 'The element of unpleasantness seems to be superimposed on a sensation which runs through the whole range.' Keele obviously finds great difficulty in describing the sensation before it becomes un-pleasant. It appears to be something more than just a pricking or burning sensation, and at one point he allows himself to talk of 'recordings of pain' at an intensity which he did not find unpleasant. Eventually he has to coin a special word 'meta-esthesia' for the range of sensation before it becomes unpleasant. His purpose is to provide us with a word which carries no connotation of pleasantness or unpleasantness. He says that the state 'metaesthesia' 'differs from true pain which by definition is always unpleasant'.

Professor A. Forbes[2] uses as example the gentle pressing of a skin surface with a finger-nail. He says that while the most gentle contact evokes only touch sensation there is soon a sharply defined change in the quality of the sensation. At this point he gets into difficulties over what to call the new sensation, which is not at first unpleasant. He says: 'The first onset (threshold) of the new (pain) sensation is very definite—an easily recognized end point. The transition to a degree of stimulation which is unpleasant, and therefore called "pain", is gradual and ill-defined.' Professor Forbes assumes that pain must be unpleasant, but he is obviously tempted to call the sensation 'pain' even when it is pleasant or neutral. He com-promises, and does use the word 'pain' but encloses it in brackets.

Any arbitrary ruling that pain is by definition unpleasant

---

[1] *The Assessment of Pain in Man and Animals* (ed. Keele and Smith), p. 30.
[2] Quoted by H. K. Beecher, *Measurement of Subjective Responses*, p. 158.

may do justice to the normal use of the word, but it will leave us powerless to describe abnormal or unusual phenomena. The sensation and our reaction to it must be differentiated, within the concept of pain, if we are to make any sense of the results of the experiments we have just been considering. Without the concept of a pain-quality all we could do would be to talk inaccurately of a 'prick', coin a new word, or timidly put the word 'pain' in brackets. With the concept, the results of the experiments seem less bewildering. We merely have examples of the quality without the normal reaction. There are very compelling grounds for asserting this. The subjects in the experiments are not just tempted to use the word 'pain' because of the similarity of the sensation to undoubted 'pains' which they had felt on other occasions. The sensation, which they wish to call 'pain', but which is not unpleasant, feels exactly the same, when it becomes unpleasant a few moments later. Yet everyone agrees that at the latter stage it can be called a 'pain'.

2. *An Analysis of Pain*

Faced with phenomena like those we have been considering, some physiologists make their own attempts to analyse pain. A marked tendency is to make 'unpleasantness' into a third element in pain, alongside the sensation and the emotional response. The best recent example of this approach occurs in a paper on 'Pain Thresholds and Analgesic Agents',[1] and a detailed examination of it may expose its error. The authors are quite ready to talk of 'pain' when it is not unpleasant. They say: 'Noxious stimulation at intensities in the range required for assessment of the absolute sensory threshold for pain evokes *only* the discriminative *sensory* aspects of pain, since stimulation in this range is neither pleasant nor unpleasant.' They define the sensory aspects of pain as being 'those features that are neither pleasant nor unpleasant, but merely furnish discriminative information—the presence of pain, its point of origin, time of onset etc.' These features form one of what they consider are the four major components of the total pain experience, namely 'simple sensation, arousal, anguish, and emotional response'. Clearly the main 'sensory aspect' of pain must be pain-quality. Unless the presence or absence of some such quality provides

[1] Chapman, Dingman and Ginzberg, *Brain*, 88 (1965), 1011–22.

the basis for the grouping of some sensations as pains and the dismissal of others because they are not, we would have no grounds for talking of 'pain' when we do not find the sensation unpleasant. How could we distinguish a pain from other sensations, if it had no distinctive feature? Every reference by the authors to the presence of *pain*, the point of origin of *pain*, or the time of onset of *pain*, presupposes (since no attempt is made to tie pain conceptually to dislike) that pain is a distinctive sensation with its own quality. If they think that the 'simple sensation' has anything less than what we mean by 'pain-quality', they cannot apply the word 'pain' to it. How far they realize this is questionable, since what they call 'the anguish components' appear to have some of the characteristics of pain-quality. They distinguish between these and the emotional components as follows:

The *anguish* components are the 'hurtful' aspects of pain—the modality-specific qualities of unpleasantness and discomfort. The *emotional* components are those highly integrated, complex, affective responses (suffering, fear, depression, anxiety, anger, humiliation, shame, etc.) to the modality-specific features of pain. Defined in this way, they are not related directly and exclusively to pain *per se*, but are more generalised reactions to its symbolic significance.

How far can this distinction be upheld? Pain can certainly be the occasion for a variety of emotions, with a variety of 'objects', and one of the most common is anxiety at its significance. In what way, however, are these to be distinguished from the anguish components'? How is the unpleasantness of a pain to be distinguished from the suffering the pain brings? It is clear that the writers of the paper view unpleasantness and discomfort as being in some way 'in' the pain. They are 'aspects' of the sensation, which disappear when it is of low intensity or affected by drugs. They are 'qualities' of the pain, and are 'modality-specific'. This presumably means that they are peculiar to pain. The emotions, on the other hand, are our responses to the pain, although the pain *per se* need not be their 'object'.

By talking of the 'sensory aspects of pain', the authors have already implicitly, if not explicitly, acknowledged a specific pain-quality. It looks as if their 'anguish-components' are additional pain-qualities over and above the basic one. They must be claiming that there is one quality for all pain, including that which is not unpleasant, and special qualities for pain which is unpleasant. It cannot be that the former is replaced by the latter when, for example, pain reaches the unpleasant stage after the application of chemicals on a blister base. It is because there are great similarities between sensations at each stage that we give the name 'pain' to both. If the quality of a sensation changed markedly when it became unpleasant, it would be easy to apply one name to it before the change and another after it, since the second stage would really be a new sensation. The writers must consider that the 'hurtful aspects' of pain are not the most distinctive part of the sensation. If they were, they would surely provide the basis on which they grouped such sensations, and gave them a common name.

In fact, not only are they not distinctive, but we might wonder if they exist at all. To have the 'quality of unpleasantness' is simply to be unpleasant. The unpleasantness of a pain is just its propensity to be disliked, because of its quality or intensity. It is not itself another quality. As we saw at the end of Chapter II, the same applies to 'discomfort', although it is an inappropriate word to use in connection with pain. Discomfort is just what we find uncomfortable. If there are 'hurtful aspects' of pain over and above pain-quality, whether they are called qualities of 'unpleasantness', 'discomfort', or something else, they must be logically distinct from our dislike. If it is analytic that such qualities or aspects are disliked, and must be present when we dislike pain and absent when we do not, it is difficult to see that we are asserting anything more, when we say that we feel them, than that we dislike the sensation of pain of which they purport to be qualities. If, on the other hand, they can be distinguished from our dislike of the pain, then it must at least be logically possible to feel a pain with the so-called qualities of unpleasantness and discomfort, and not dislike it. In that case, they have been wrongly named. They may be distinctive varieties of pain, but they have no intrinsic link with unpleasantness. Mention of them does not necessarily involve any reference to our dislike of the pain. It just tells us what kind of pain it is.

The authors of the paper are the victims of the belief that if we dislike a sensation which we formerly did not find unpleasant, or if we no longer mind one which we formerly disliked, then the sensation itself must have changed. As we saw in Chapter V, it need not have. By the same argument, it could be maintained that if there are 'qualities of unpleasantness', and if they are not necessarily disliked, the sensation must have a special quality when we do dislike them, to explain our dislike on that occasion. We could then raise the question whether it was analytic that the special quality was disliked, and the same problems as we have just dealt with would arise concerning the 'quality of unpleasantness'. It is surely more reasonable to admit that the sensation could remain the same in quality while our attitude to it changes.

If the 'anguish' components of the pain experience are anything besides the pain-quality or the qualities of different species of pain, they can only be our reaction to the pain-quality. If they are not the components of the 'total pain experience' which give us anguish, then they must be that anguish. In that case, they are not very different from the 'suffering', which the authors admit is one of the 'emotional components'. In connection with pain, 'suffering' implies distress or a high degree of dislike. To ask if someone suffered much as a result of the pain of a disease is to ask whether he was distressed or whether he found it exceptionally unpleasant. One of the authors' four components in the 'total pain experience' cannot therefore be distinguished from what they include in another. Within the group of the emotional components we must distinguish between the emotions which take the pain *per se* as their 'object' and those which take its significance, but that is the only ground of distinction.

The authors also claim that there is a fourth element in the 'total pain experience'. They point both to the effect of drugs and to that of certain brain operations, which, unlike leucotomy, do not influence the emotions. After 'thalamotomy', they say, 'when queried about their pain, the patients reported that it could still be perceived, if an effort was made to focus their attention on it; distraction occurred spontaneously'. It is concluded from this that 'they are relieved of the features of the total pain experience, related to tension, arousal, and domination of attention'. It looks as if the authors are making the same mistake as they made with the 'anguish components'. Just as they thought that the pain must have a specific quality to explain our dislike of it, so they appear to assume that if we are absorbed in the pain, it must have a distinctive feature to explain our absorption. If the pain does not demand our attention, then even though, if we make an effort to pay attention to it, we may still recognize the sensation as pain, the special feature of the experience must have gone. It is difficult to see what is added by talking about this mysterious feature. If it is only present when our attention is drawn to the pain, what need have we to say anything more than that our attention is drawn to the pain? The authors seem to have a causal model in mind. They say: 'The arousal components are concerned with altering alarm, tension, and domination of attention.' They seem to be claiming that we feel the arousal components of the experience. Their insistence that they are parts of the 'total pain experience' suggests this. When we feel them our attention is dominated as a result. Their use of the words 'alarm' and 'tension' is presumably intended to provide rough synonyms for the 'domination of our attention', but it merely confuses matters because of their connections with 'fear' and 'anxiety', which are very definitely part of the emotional components.

It is perhaps significant that there is no normal word in ordinary language to refer to these 'arousal components' which suddenly disappear at the highly notional point at which we no longer find our attention demanded but have to make an effort to pay it. The concept which is relevant here is that of intensity. The patients who found that distraction from their pain occurred spontaneously could not have had a very severe pain. In fact it must have been a very moderate one, although, if they were completely preoccupied with the pain *per se* before the operation, it was then very severe. The operation must have reduced the intensity of the pain. It has not taken away a feature of the experience which was present before. The pain does not cease to have intensity, when it stops demanding attention. Its intensity just diminishes, since it is logically impossible for a pain to have none. Such a pain would be like a 'pain which does not exist'. It would not be a pain at all. The reason is clear if we remember the conceptual link with attention. A pain with no intensity would be a pain to which we paid no attention, and such a pain would be one which we did not feel. The paying of attention, whether it is demanded or not, is a necessary condition for the feeling of *all* pain, even the pain of low intensity which is usually neither pleasant nor unpleasant.

3. *The Enjoyment of Suffering*

We have concentrated so far on the possibility of 'non-painful' pain. If, however, a sensation can have pain-quality without being disliked, is it logically possible that it be positively liked? Clearly this is so. Only if we already dislike something is there a logical bar to liking it. It is self-contradictory both to like and dislike something at the same time, for the same reasons, although we can like some features and dislike others which belong to the same object. It follows that I cannot dislike a sensation of pain *per se* and at the same time like it *per se*. It is possible to dislike a pain for its own sake, and yet to be overjoyed at its significance, as, for example, when it is a sign that one's back is not broken. It would not be logically possible to be overjoyed at that pain for its own sake while we still disliked it. That would be to welcome and to wish to be rid of the same thing at the same time for the same reason. If the 'object', the time, or the ground of our joy was different from that of our dislike, there would be no contradiction.

The way in which many people apparently enjoy searching with their tongue for a tooth which aches slightly, and deliberately try to manipulate it, might confirm that it is quite intelligible to like pain. Their liking for low degrees of pain would explain their deliberate attempts to aggravate the ache. Whether this is the right explanation, it is surely a possible one. The major examples of apparent enjoyment of pain, however, occur in the phenomenon of masochism. It is often assumed that the masochist simultaneously dislikes and enjoys pain. It seems as if for the same reason he both wants to be rid of the pain and wants it to continue. If it is also thought that pain is necessarily disliked, the phenomenon becomes bewildering. Freud says[1]:

If mental processes are governed by the pleasure principle in such a way that their first aim is the avoidance of unpleasure and the obtaining of pleasure, masochism is incomprehensible. If pain and unpleasure be not simply warnings but actually aims, the pleasure principle is paralysed.

[1] 'The Economic Problem of Masochism', Standard Ed. 19, 159–70.

Freud takes physical pain to be a particular case of 'un-pleasure'. It is thus by definition the opposite of pleasure, and his usual description of 'primary' masochism as being 'pleasure in pain' apparently becomes a straight contradiction. This can be avoided if we resist the temptation of thinking that physical pain need necessarily be connected with 'unpleasure'. It is merely a usual 'object' of unpleasure. *Mental* pain is 'unpleasure', and the question must be raised whether it is logically possible to seek this for its own sake. I may endure personal distress and anguish for what I conceive as being a desirable end. If, however, someone says: 'I want to suffer' and gives as his only reason the fact that he likes suffering for its own sake, would we have to conclude that he was using the word 'suffering' in an eccentric way, and that he does not mean the same by it as we do? This is a separate point from the fact that what distresses him may be very different from what distresses us. He may for example be unmoved at a great per-sonal tragedy, or be very agitated at some trivial occurrence, when for instance anyone walked on a lawn (perhaps because he thought that the blades of grass had feelings). In each case we could sensibly talk of his 'distress' or lack of it, even though our own emotional reactions to similar situations may be unlike his in every way. His view of the situation and his agitation (or lack of it) would give us the clue to his emotional state.

If someone is definitely distressed and suffering, is there any logical contradiction in saying that he is enjoying it and wants his state of misery to continue? Can it really be 'misery' he is feeling, if he does not want to be rid of it? Certainly he must want to be rid of the 'object' of his distress. He cannot both be distressed at a pain and want it to go on. If he did not want it relieved, he could not 'really' be distressed at it. Granted, however, that someone wants to be rid of the 'object' of his distress, is it a part of the concept of suffering that he should want his suffering (or distress) to leave him? The answer to this question might be relevant to the primary form of masochism (which involves actual physical pain), if masochists do dislike the pain they appear to seek. It is certainly relevant to what Freud and his successors call 'moral masochism'. This term is applied to individuals who apparently show a marked tendency in their lives to seek out situations which give them suffering and mental pain. Freud says of them[1]: 'The suffering itself is what matters: whether it is decreed by someone who is loved or by someone who is indifferent is of no importance. ... The true masochist always turns his cheek, whenever he has a chance of receiving a blow.' Elsewhere[2] Freud talks of those 'who find their pleasure, not in having *physical* pain inflicted on them, but in humiliation and mental torture'. The theory is complicated by the fact that the pleasure, which Freud thinks is sexual, is also unconscious. Moral masochists do not consciously seek out suffering for its own sake, and do not admit to enjoying it. In this they differ from masochists who seek physical pain. Indeed the only reason Freud appears to have for talking of pleasure in this connection is that some people do appear to seek out distressing situations. The fact that they would deny that they were doing anything of the sort might make us uneasy about this. If one believes that people do seek only pleasure, it must be very tempting to stipulate that if they seek suffering they must be enjoying it, and this is what Freud at times appears to be doing. The regularity with which someone finds himself in distressing situations is not by itself a sufficient reason for a psycho-analyst to claim that the person is really seeking them out because he enjoys them. The man's denial that this is so is not completely convincing, as it is always possible that he is the victim of self-deception. It must be reinforced by an absence of any signs of enjoyment of any possible good aspect of the situation. If, for instance, he has a quickened step, a brightened eye, and an obvious feeling of self-importance in the midst of his troubles, we might suspect that for some reason he really relished them. If, however, his whole demeanour and view of the situation is obviously one of utter distress, it is implausible to insist that he is unconsciously enjoying it.

Even if it is possible to betray signs of enjoyment in a distressing situation, can the distress itself be the 'object' of the enjoyment? I can certainly enjoy one thing, and at the same time suffer because of another. Even here, there would probably be a clash, with one mood predominating over the other. Can I actually enjoy the suffering? I may regard it as a penance, and rejoice in the fact that I am suffering, but this would not be to

[1] 'The Economic Problem of Masochism', Standard Ed. 19, p. 165.
[2] Standard Ed. 4, 159.

take joy in the suffering itself, for its own sake. If the suffering itself was the 'object', the more I suffered, or the more I was distressed, the more I would enjoy it. Similarly if the pleasure I took in something was the 'object' of my distress, the more I enjoyed whatever it was, the more I would suffer. Here again this is different from being distressed at *the fact that* I am enjoying it. I might for example think that I was enjoying something that was morally wrong. I might enjoy seeing the suffering of others and be very distressed at my sadism. The degree of my enjoyment would not necessarily influence the degree of my distress in this instance. The fact that I am even enjoying the situation a little might distress me a great deal. On the other hand, if the enjoyment itself was the 'object', there would be a close correlation between the two, so that I could take a great deal of enjoyment in something, and at the same time be highly distressed. As the enjoyment was itself the 'object' and ground of my distress, it would obviously be the main factor in influencing it.

It does seem highly paradoxical for suffering and enjoyment to march together in this way, but it is not obviously self-contradictory. If I was distressed at physical pain, and enjoyed my distress, my enjoyment and my distress would apparently be at different levels, with different 'objects'. There seems to be no question of finding the same thing both pleasant and unpleasant. I find the pain unpleasant and my distress pleasant. In other words I would want the pain to stop and the distress to continue. This is different from the self-contradictory position of the person who both enjoyed and was distressed by the pain *per se*, although there are similarities. In both cases, the enjoyment is dependent on the continuance of the pain. In the one, the pain is simply what I enjoy. In the other, I enjoy my distress at the pain. In each instance, once the pain stops, so do my enjoyment and my distress.

If someone wants his pain to stop and his distress at that pain to continue, it is logically impossible that he satisfy both his desires. If he is freed of his pain, as he wishes, his distress will vanish with its 'object'. This in turn, however, deprives his enjoyment of its 'object', and he can no longer enjoy what he wants to. If the latter desire is satisfied and his distress continues, this presupposes that the pain remains despite his desire to be rid of it. To enjoy his distress, he would have both to want his pain to continue as the 'object' of his distress, and want it to stop precisely because it is the 'object' of that distress. There is no logical impossibility in having conflicting desires. It is all too common a phenomenon to want to have one's cake and at the same time to want to eat it. This is to be distinguished from wanting what is logically impossible. I cannot want a situation in which I have the cake and do not have it. That is to desire a position that logically could not occur. Wanting p and not-p is different from wanting p and wanting not-p. In the first case, I desire a logically impossible situation, and therefore the desire is itself logically impossible. In the second, I desire two perfectly possible situations, but the simultaneous satisfaction of my desires is logically impossible. It is, however, logically possible for me to have the desires simultaneously. This would suggest that it is completely intelligible to want a pain to continue at the same time as wanting it to stop. It might therefore be possible to enjoy distress at pain. Nevertheless, as the satisfaction of both desires is impossible, it would be natural for one to gain the upper hand. My distress might become so great that I might want to be rid of the pain more than anything else. If, however, my enjoyment increased with my distress, I might also want my distress (and hence the pain) to continue more than anything else. It can be seen that in this extreme case each desire leaves no room for the other. I logically cannot have two desires, each stronger than the other.

If high degrees of pleasure and distress conflict logically, can we still accept that it is possible, if highly abnormal, to enjoy moderate degrees of distress? It is immediately clear that not all circumstances in which enjoyment and distress are linked are cases where one is the 'object' of the other. We have already seen that one can enjoy the fact that one is distressed, and that this is different from the enjoyment of distress. It must also be possible to enjoy the expression of distress or the feelings associated with it without actually enjoying being distressed. I could like giving vent to my feelings without in any way liking the occasion of those feelings. Some people are said to 'luxuriate in their grief' or simply to 'have a good cry', and to do this they need not relish the 'object' of their grief. Their grief could be genuine and unforced, but they could still enjoy 'letting themselves go'. This would be particularly true in countries where the uninhibited public display of grief is the convention. Similarly, I could enjoy giving vent to my distress without wanting the 'object' of my emotion to continue and without welcoming it in any way. My enjoyment could be betrayed by the abandoned way I gave expression to my emotion, and my disinclination to control myself, although this need not cast doubt on the reality of my distress. I could still be highly pleased to discover that the 'object' of my distress was only imaginary.

It is also possible to enjoy the feelings which are associated with an emotion. Presumably people go to see horror films because they enjoy feeling frightened. Whether they could enjoy actually being frightened in a real situation of terror is another matter. In the same way, it should be logically possible to enjoy feeling distressed, that is to say, to enjoy the feelings one usually has when one is distressed. I could do this without enjoying being distressed, and I would presumably be only too pleased if I could have the feelings without the unpleasant context. In that case, I would just be enjoying thrills or pangs, and not thrills 'of fear', or pangs 'of distress'.

We have emphasized that enjoyment of distress must be distinguished from enjoyment of the fact that one is distressed, enjoyment of the expression of distress, and enjoyment of the feelings of distress. We might well wonder what is left, and it is remarkably difficult to find an example of enjoyment of distress which does not somehow collapse into one of these three. We have seen that enjoyment of distress must involve a desire for the distress (and hence the 'object' of our distress) to be continued. It involves seeing the distress as in some way good in itself. There must be something about it that we like. The difficulty is that it seems impossible to explain what this could be. The clash of wants which we uncovered in the hypothetical situation of enjoying distress is itself symptomatic of the basic incoherence of the position. How can I view the viewing of something as bad as itself good? I may enjoy some aspect of the experience—perhaps the feelings attached to it. I may relish the fact that I become disturbed and distressed at something because it shows that I am sensitive and highly moral. I may obtain a good deal of pleasure in giving vent to my emotion (and perhaps becoming the object of sympathy). All these are possibilities which we have considered, and distinguished from the actual enjoyment of distress. It can be no accident that every combination of pleasure and distress turns out to be different from enjoyment of distress. It must be that the total experience of being distressed is not in itself the kind of thing which we can find pleasant. It would indeed be very strange if the process of finding something unpleasant could itself be pleasant. There would be a fundamental clash between our view of the situation as bad for us in some way and our view of the same situation with a few extras as good for us in some way. If we are told that it is the extras which make the difference, we are probably being taken back to the position that what is being enjoyed is the fact that we are distressed, our feelings of distress, or our expression of our emotion.

4. *The Enjoyment of Pain*

If all this is correct, it is a dangerous simplification to talk as if masochists enjoy *suffering*. The word 'suffering' implies the presence of distress, and we have agreed that it is logically impossible to enjoy this. The most plausible candidate to be the 'object' of masochistic enjoyment in a combination of enjoyment and suffering might well be 'the fact that one is suffering'. The masochist could well enjoy the significance of the suffering. If the suffering represented punishment for him and he desired punishment (for suitable psychological reasons), the situation at once becomes more intelligible. The experience of suffering would not itself be important. What it meant to the masochist might well be.

We have concentrated so far on whether a masochist can enjoy suffering or distress, although we have asserted that pain could logically be enjoyed. There are many philosophers who would cast doubt on the intelligibility of enjoying pain, usually out of a desire to define pain as a 'sensation which is disliked'. Certainly enjoyment of pain must be parasitic on the normal link between a sensation of pain and dislike. Otherwise, as we have seen, the concept of pain could never be taught. Someone who merely claims to 'enjoy pain' would make us suspect that he did not really understand what pain was, unless he gave us evidence that he did by frequently using the word normally. Even if he talked of pain in circumstances where we would expect him to feel it, it might still be open for us to conclude that he was not feeling pain at all if he showed no sign of dislike. He would have had to have given proof that he had learnt the concept properly, by using, at least at some period in his life, the word 'pain' of sensations he obviously disliked.

It is therefore of considerable importance that the masochist apparently only enjoys certain pains in certain circumstances. He usually uses the word 'pain' perfectly normally. If, for example, he broke his leg, he would show signs of distress and talk of pain in a perfectly normal manner. Sandor Ferenczi says[1]:

I have it on the authority of an extremely intelligent young man who suffered from this perversion that each masochist finds pleasure only in a special degree of humiliation and bodily suffering to which the partner in each case is specially enjoined to conform.

The situation seems to be one in which someone gives ample evidence of his grasp of the concept, and yet suddenly uses the word 'pain' in an eccentric way on a few specific occasions. Only a rigid belief in the logical impropriety of failing to dislike 'pain' would make anyone dismiss them out of hand as possible instances of feeling pain. It would seem more reasonable to assume that they are merely examples of feeling pain, but reacting to it in an abnormal way. Kenny claims[2]: 'Since the masochist's reaction to his sensation is not a pain-reaction, the only reason that we have for calling it "pain" is that it is caused by treatment which from other men elicits pain-reactions.' In fact, the masochist's own inclination to call what he feels 'pain', coupled with his normally correct use of the word, is our only guide. A reliance on the cause could land us in trouble. What, after all, if an apparent masochist was in fact congenitally insensitive to pain? The cause might be one which almost universally results in pain, but would not in this particular case.

We have concluded that it is perfectly intelligible for a masochist to enjoy a sensation of pain. On the other hand, he could not enjoy suffering, but only something such as the fact that he was suffering. Is either of these possibilities the correct description? Do masochists merely feel pain without disliking it, or do they find it positively unpleasant at the same time as they gain

---

[1] *Further Contributions to the Theory and Technique of Psycho-Analysis*, p. 280.
[2] *Action, Emotion and Will*, p. 118.

some kind of pleasure from the significance of the situation? It seems that masochists both admit to feeling pain, and show signs of distress. It looks as if we can rule out the possibility of masochists enjoying the sensation of pain. If they exhibit pain-behaviour, they must be disliking the sensation *per se*. It is nevertheless true that they do seek out the sensation, and do not try to be rid of it when they do feel it. Despite their dislike of it, they are clearly enduring it for the sake of something else (presumably sexual pleasure). Indeed the chairman of a symposium[1] on the subject of masochism claimed that the term 'masochism' 'should be employed only when pain and unpleasure occur as the necessary conditions for sexual gratifi-cations'. Pain may be the cause of pleasure, but it is not itself the 'object' of any pleasure. There may be exceptions to this rule, but the distinction between cause and 'object' is itself sufficient to clear away many of the contradictions which were apparently inherent in masochism. J. Hospers[2] distinguishes two senses of pleasure, one (pleasure$_1$) the opposite of 'dis-pleasure', the other (pleasure$_2$) the opposite of the sensation of pain. He uses the first in connection with masochism, and says of the masochist:

How could he take pleasure in the opposite of pleasure, pain? But in fact there is no puzzle at all: the infliction of pain on his body *causes* him (for reasons familiar to psychoanalysts) to experience pleasure$_1$, whereas such pain causes most persons displeasure. . . . The infliction of the pain is precisely what gives him the pleasure. To say that pain is pleasant sounds paradoxical: but the paradox disappears when we distinguish the double sense of 'pleasure'.

We have examined the 'double sense' of 'pleasure' in Chapter VI. It is sufficient here to draw attention to the fact that to say that pain is pleasant is not necessarily to say that pain *causes* pleasure. 'Objects' are often also the causes of emotion, but they need not be (although, of course, all emotions must have 'objects'). If I say that a pain is pleasant, I might merely mean that I found it pleasant, that I took pleasure in it. The cause of this might be one of the reasons 'familiar to psycho-analysts' and not the pain. It is very easy to slide from talking about 'objects' to talking about causes. Hospers does it when he says that

[1] Reported by M. H. Stein, *J. American Psychoanalytical Association*, 4 (1956), 526–38.   [2] *Human Conduct*, p. 113.

the infliction of pain on a masochist 'gives him the pleasure'. This harmless phrase could mean that it is what the masochist takes pleasure in (and this is to talk about an 'object'). It could also mean that the infliction of pain *causes* him pleasure, and if this sense is confused with the previous one we are deprived of any possibility of distinguishing a necessary condition for pleasure from the actual 'object' of that pleasure. The cause must then also be the 'object'. This assumption creates many complications, as the casual connection between pain and pleasure in the phenomenon of masochism is not in doubt (although psycho-analysts freely admit that they do not know how the two become associated.) What is very questionable is whether masochists actually take pleasure in the pain, or whether they treat it merely as an essential means to pleasure.

The references of psycho-analysts to masochism contain many examples of the blurring of the distinction between cause and 'object'. It looks as if masochists dislike pain, and yet as a result of it gain sexual satisfaction. What they take pleasure in, therefore, are sexual sensations, and these are mysteriously caused by pain. The pain is not itself pleasurable, although it may causally be the source of their pleasure. Yet, in the symposium already quoted, R. M. Loewenstein says[1]: 'Perversion is characterised by a special capacity to experience pain as pleasurable.' Is he putting forward the thesis that the masochist does after all actually enjoy *pain*? It would appear not, as he goes on to claim: 'The moral masochist derives no sexual pleasure from suffering as the pervert does.' It looks as if he regards suffering as the mere cause of sexual pleasure. Certainly pain could not be the 'object' of such pleasure, which is merely a particular class of sensation. As such, it would itself be a candidate as an 'object' of some emotion-like member of the concept of pleasure.

Another contributor to the symposium, Ludwig Eidelberg, is reported as saying 'The masochistic pervert accepts punishment and approves of it, while the moral masochist denies his need of it, and insists that his suffering is purely accidental.' We have agreed that for this very reason talk of 'pleasure' in connection with the phenomenon of moral masochism is dubious. In the perversion proper the masochist does consciously

---

[1] *J. American Psychoanalytic Association*, 4 (1956), 530.

seek pain. Eidelberg sees this as an apparent contradiction of the 'pleasure-unpleasure principle' and says: 'The
masochist appears to seek unpleasure for its own sake.' He
also claims: 'The masochist really craves unpleasure, and should
be so diagnosed only if he pursues aims which are experienced
unpleasant by himself.' It is, however, strange only if the
masochist seeks 'unpleasure' as an end in itself. If he just wants
it because it is a necessary condition for his obtaining sexual
gratification, it is not odd at all. Presumably if he could obtain
satisfaction without suffering, he would do so. Something in his
psychological make-up means that this is impossible for him.
Eidelberg himself talks of the pervert accepting punishment
'only as a condition' for sexual pleasure, and if he admits this,
it is difficult to see why he should be so puzzled about the
apparent desire for unpleasure. The masochist 'approves' of it
only as a means to an end. It is significant that he 'approves'
only of suffering which is controlled by himself. Masochists are,
if anything, more frightened than normal people of suffering
which is outside their control. Such suffering does not serve
their purposes. This is surely an indication that they do not
desire suffering for its own sake, but that they want only the
particular kind of suffering in a setting which gives them the
required result. Just because their suffering is a cause of their
pleasure (or rather of sensations which they take pleasure in), it
need not be the 'object' of that pleasure.

In *Masochism in Modern Man* T. Reik agrees with this interpretation. He says[1]: 'The punishment or humiliation precedes
the satisfaction. The pleasurable excitement they awaken is
only apparently and indirectly concerned with pain and shame.
In reality it is aimed at the following anticipated satisfaction.'
He claims[2]: 'The discomfort is not desired as such, but it constitutes the price of pleasure.' 'Discomfort', of course, could not
logically be desired for its own sake. If one finds a position or
situation uncomfortable, amongst other things one wants to get
out of it. It is logically impossible to want to get into a situation
for its own sake at the same time as one wants to get out of it for
the same reason. Reik's basic point, however, does hold
good. A masochist does not delight in situations which
normal people find uncomfortable. He too dislikes them, but

[1] p. 269.   [2] p. 123.

endures them for the sake of pleasure which they causally produce.

Reik admits there are complications. Although he emphasizes that discomfort and pain 'are merely the indispensable condition for attaining sexual satisfaction',[1] he does say[2]: 'Ultimately the conscious boundaries become indistinct: the discomfort, the pain and the humiliation themselves become pleasure.' Similarly he says[3]: 'Finally pleasure edges into discomfort itself.' His use of a phrase such as 'pain becomes pleasure' makes the process sound very mysterious. Presumably he means that it becomes pleasurable, rather than that the pain itself changes to something else. If the sensation did change (and it could), there would not even be a ghost of a conceptual problem left, because the masochist would have no inclination to talk of 'pain'. What causes pain in others would not cause any in him. Reik's grouping of such disparate concepts as those of pain, discomfort and humiliation also clouds the issue. Is he saying that a 'sophisticated' masochist comes to like sensations which he originally disliked or found uncomfortable or which were produced in humiliating circumstances? Might he on the other hand mean that such a masochist begins to enjoy the fact that he is suffering, finding something uncomfortable, or being humiliated, because these sensations come to be linked in his mind with gaining pleasure? His reference to pain might suggest the former, while his reference to humiliation might indicate the latter. If the sophisticated masochist shows signs of dislike and distress, but claims that he is enjoying something besides the sexual pleasure he derives from the situation, the latter interpretation is presumably the correct one. The alternatives may each be psychologically abnormal, perhaps even by masochistic standards. We have seen that they are both logically possible.

[1] *Masochism in Modern Man*, p. 308.   [2] p. 122.   [3] p. 123.

IX

CONGENITAL INSENSITIVITY
TO PAIN

1. *A Case of Insensitivity to Pain*

WE have analysed the concept of the quality of sensations in a
different way from that of their intensity. Sensations are
classified on the basis of their quality, and names such as 'pain'
are given to the more distinctive types. Because of this the way
someone describes his sensations must be conclusive. He might
himself have second thoughts about the description which he
has used, but it is not open to anybody else to contradict him.
The only proviso is that we must be satisfied that he has learnt
what the concept of pain is. Those who have tried to tie the
sensation of pain to dislike have attempted to provide us with
public criteria in the shape of expressions of dislike. Because one
can dislike sensations which everyone would deny were pains,
and not dislike sensations which are said to be pains, this
attempt must be dismissed. A sensation of pain is logically
distinct from our dislike of it.

In contrast with this, we have not insisted that those who feel a
pain are in a privileged position when it comes to judging its
intensity. We have placed intensity in the same kind of category
as dislike, rather than as pain-quality. Someone who lies in
bed in a perfectly contented manner without the slightest
inclination to cry out or to show any other sign of finding any
sensation unpleasant could hardly be said to dislike pain, if he
was feeling it. Similarly we have maintained that someone who
was able to ignore pain easily, when he felt it, and gave no
evidence of being distracted, could hardly be said to be
suffering intense pain. It is as much a conceptual truth that
intense pain demands our attention, as that dislike of a sensation
involves at least an inclination to wince, moan, or indulge in
other appropriate behaviour. Intensity is not to be treated as
another quality in sensations. We do not say that sensations are
'the same kind' merely because they are of the same intensity.

A growth of intensity does not mean that one feature of a sensation becomes accentuated. The whole sensation, with whatever qualities it has, becomes more noticeable.

Because intensity has such a firm behavioural link, even someone who had been numb from birth would be able to understand something of what intensity in sensations was. He would have no difficulty in associating it with a demand on attention. Such a person would, however, find it very hard to differentiate between sensations other than by distinguishing various types of reaction. Even if he was able to grasp the concept of a sensation, he would not be able to understand what the quality of a sensation was, because of the lack of a firm logical link which would invariably bind it to publicly observable phenomena. He would by observation be able to associate pain with bodily injury, and he would realize that it was an unpleasant sensation. He would not be able to distinguish between a situation where the same sensation was felt and not disliked, and where it was not felt. All talk of 'the same sensation' must for him involve reference to a similar reaction. Pains would be sensations which evoke manifestations of dislike. He could not think of them as being similar in any other respect. As a result he would not grasp the possibility of pains which were not unpleasant, or unpleasant sensations which were not pains. If he was told that a pain was not merely an unpleasant sensation, he would be unable to understand what a 'pain' was. Anyone who was not numb but was congenitally insensitive to pain might well be in a similar position.

There are several reports in the literature of physiology concerning patients who have shown greater or lesser degrees of apparent insensitivity to pain. They were not numb. They could distinguish between hot and cold, and could also tell when they were subjected to a pin-prick. It appears, however, that they did not feel pains. Their experiences in situations which would produce pain in normal people strongly suggested this. They showed no signs of dislike or distress, and said that they felt no particularly distinctive kind of sensation. The following report is typical[1]:

The patient said that six days previously he had inadvertently held his left hand in a gas flame, while heating glue, but when he saw

[1] E. C. Jewsbury, *Brain*, 74 (1951), 339.

this, he felt no discomfort, and was aware only of a tingling sensation in the fingers.

Is such a person feeling pain without disliking it, or not feeling pain at all? Is this case like the case of asymbolia for pain, which we encountered, in which pain was felt and not disliked? As the abnormality is congenital, we are unable to rely on the patient's grasp of the concept of pain, as shown in his previous normal use of pain vocabulary. It follows that we must always be suspicious about reports or denials of pain which are made by someone who is apparently congenitally insensitive to pain. He has *ex hypothesi* given no previous evidence of feeling pain, and has never reported pain in normal circumstances. There has never been an opportunity to teach him, through his own experience, what pain was, or to find out from his own reports of pain in appropriate circumstances that he had learnt the concept correctly.

There is therefore some plausibility in holding that those who are apparently insensitive to pain are merely indifferent to it. They feel what would normally be called pain, but do not dislike it. The 'tingling sensation' felt by the patient was really 'pain'. We have agreed that this situation is logically possible. Even, however, if the man had never learnt to call the 'tingling sensation' 'pain', he would surely realize that he was feeling the same sensation in a variety of circumstances. If the different kinds of pain have any quality in common, as we have maintained, we would expect the quality to be recognized even by those who did not find it unpleasant. The reports of congenital insensitivity to pain made by physiologists do not suggest that this happens. Not only do patients deny feeling a distinctive sensation, but they are very prone to injury. If they felt pain but did not dislike it, we would expect them to learn through experience that the distinctive sensation which they sometimes felt was often a sign of bodily damage. If the man who held his hand in a gas flame had felt pain, we ought to find that it served as a warning to him. The fact that he took no particular notice of the 'tingling sensation' might indicate that that was all it was. It must also be significant that he was not numb, and presumably possessed a normal vocabulary for sensations other than pains. He ought, then, to understand the difference between tingles and other types of sensation. If he said that the sensation was a tingle, why should we think otherwise?

The reason some physiologists claim that there is no such thing as insensitivity to pain lies in their conception of what 'pain' is. They assume that pain is merely an 'unpleasant sensation'. For them any sensation combined with distress or dislike is by definition a pain. We have already come across those who believe that the ability to feel a pin-prick normally is a satisfactory indication not just that a patient is not numb, but that he can feel pain. Their assumption is that our adverse attitude to the sensation provides all that is distinctive in pain. It follows that in cases of 'congenital insensitivity' to pain where the patients are not numb, all that is missing is the attitude. The sensation itself would be merely one of pressure, cutting, heat or something similar. That, however, is all a sensation of pain ever is. According to this view, if our attitude to the sensation changes while the sensation remains the same, we would have to say that the sensation was no longer a pain. It is significant that to say that a sensation which was a pain is so no longer is usually considered to be a remark about the sensation, and not our attitude.

There are comprehensive reports in the literature of the case of one young woman who, it seems, did not feel any pain at all for most of her life. As a result she suffered considerable physical damage regularly, and it merely went unnoticed or was regarded with indifference. Apart from this she was perfectly normal and well-balanced, and her intelligence and education made here a particularly articulate subject. Like the other cases she was not numb. She could distinguish between touch alone and touch associated with pin-prick. She could, for example, feel 'something sticking into the skin'. She could also tell the difference between hot and cold objects, even when the difference was not very great. It is interesting, however, that she said that she had never felt the sensation of itch. She is reported to have had ample opportunity to observe the behaviour of others in response to itching from such things as sunburn or chickenpox. The case-history continues[1]:

She often, simultaneously with others, had experienced the same causes for itching; yet she had never felt any particularly different

[1] G. A. McMurray, *Archives of Neurology and Psychiatry*, 64 (1950), 654.

sensation or any occasion for behaviour such as she observed in friends.

It is her lack of any feeling of pain which is most striking. We are told of the results of controlled experiments devised to test her sensitivity to pain[1]:

At no time during any of the experiments using noxious stimuli did the subject report a sensation or feeling, which could be interpreted as a report of pain. Ache, unpleasantness, unbearableness, or pain itself was never described. Consistent with this was the complete absence of any observable sign of painful experience.

Much of this would merely suggest that she did not dislike pain. It is clear, however, from the fact that she did not recognize any distinctive sensation as present in all or most of the tests to which she was subjected that she was not feeling pain. She did not feel the same sensation in one test as she felt in another, although each test would normally produce pain. It seems that she felt the kind of sensation she would have felt if she had been normal, with the element of pain subtracted. She would have a burning sensation instead of a burning pain, for example. She could not be said to be indifferent to pain, as this would suggest that she was feeling the same sensation on different occasions and never minded it. If the concept of pain-quality is disregarded, the very phrase 'indifference to pain' becomes a contradiction. The alternative to 'pain-quality' is to define pain as an unpleasant sensation. If a sensation is not unpleasant, it cannot be a 'pain'. It follows that if someone is indifferent to a sensation and does not dislike it, then it cannot be a 'pain'. The answer may come that, even if we do not dislike it on this occasion, the fact that we normally find this kind of sensation unpleasant justifies our talking of 'pain' here. What kind of sensation? One which in an important respect is the same as many other unpleasant sensations? Once we realize in addition that not all sensations which are normally unpleasant can be called 'pains', we are well on the way to formulating the concept of pain-quality as being what a certain class of normally unpleasant sensations have in common. The phrase 'indifference to pain' must imply that 'pains' have a more important similarity to each other than our normal reaction to them. Anyone who is indifferent to pain must be feeling a

[1] op. cit. p. 660.

distinctive type of sensation. The young woman whose case we are considering denied that she was. Unless we are willing to say that she is incapable of talking about her sensations at all (and she gave ample evidence to the contrary in her reports of pin-pricks, warmth and coldness and so on), we must accept this. It must have been the case that she was not feeling pain. She was insensitive to it and not merely indifferent.

2. Itches

If the concept of pain-quality plays a central part in the concept of pain, would anyone who had never felt pain fail to under-stand altogether what pain was? The young woman in question had never felt the sensation of itch, although she had experienced the usual causes of it. She had not felt any particu-larly different sensation on such occasions, and had had no desire to scratch. Would her abnormality place her in the same position with respect to itch as to pain? Is the quality of itch as important conceptually as that of pain?

There is a fundamental distinction between the concept of pain and that of itch. With the latter our reaction, namely the desire to scratch, is the major component. Indeed, to say that one has an itch and no desire to scratch is self-contradictory. If we do not in the least want to scratch, then it is merely a 'pricking sensation' or something similar. We may, of course, not want to scratch because we know we will make the condition worse, but in that situation we might still have a desire to scratch. It would merely be overridden by a longer-term desire. Scratching, or at least a desire to scratch, is so much part of the concept of itch, that it has seemed plausible to some to maintain that an itch in a certain place is just our desire to scratch that part. It is clear, however, that we do not just wish to scratch for no reason, when we have an itch. We want to scratch because of a definite kind of sensation.

It may be suggested that, as with pain, one can have a sensa-tion with 'itch-quality' without the normal reaction, and although this seems plausible, it ignores the fact that the bond which binds different kinds of 'itches' together is not so much the similarity of their 'feel' as the sameness of our reaction. 'I'm itching' and 'I want to scratch' are virtually synonymous. To emphasize the quality of the sensation is very misleading. It may be interesting to note that we feel the kind of sensation which usually makes us want to scratch, and yet that on this occasion we have no desire to do so, but it is wrong to continue to talk of 'itch' in such a context. One of the main indications which we have found of the importance of the quality of pain for the concept of pain is the fact that we do not give the name 'pain' to all sensations which we dislike. If the concept of itch ran completely parallel and the quality of the sensation was equally important (and there is no *a priori* reason why this should not be so), we would expect that there would be some sensations which would make us want to scratch, but which we would not want to call 'itches'. There do not seem to be any. A tickle, for instance, typically makes us want to brush aside whatever is irritating our skin, rather than to scratch the particular spot. An itch, therefore, happens to be defined by our reaction to the sensation and not by the quality of the sensation.

Anyone who was congenitally insensitive to pain and itch would be in a far stronger position to understand the concept of itch than that of pain simply because the quality is so much less important. They would be in no danger of relying excessively on the importance of the reaction and of underrating the significance of the quality. If they think of an itch as being a sensation which makes people want to scratch, they will always be right, whereas if they think of pain as being a distressing sensation which people try to avoid, they are conceptually mistaken. They will not understand that some pains are not disliked and that some unpleasant sensations are not pain. It is clear that it is completely within their power to understand what is meant by a 'sensation which makes people want to scratch'. They can understand what a sensation is and have sensations themselves. They can understand what scratching is and imitate others doing it. It would not require a great leap of imagination for them to put the two together. Indeed, if they are told that an itch usually feels something like a pricking sensation, they might even understand what it feels like, although, as we have seen, this is an irrelevant detail.

3. *Pain and Error*

How far in fact would those who are congenitally insensitive to pain be forced to conceive of pain as being merely an unpleasant sensation? Are they completely unable to understand the importance of the quality of pain? Will they, as a result, sometimes talk of pain wrongly in situations where someone who had a normal understanding of the concept would not dream of using the word? One of the most interesting passages in the case-history of the young woman concerns a belief which she had that she was beginning to feel pain. It says[1]:

There was evidence of a curiosity as to what feeling could produce the pronounced pain reaction she has observed in others. She also expressed the belief, that, to a large extent, her sensitivity to painful stimuli was increasing. This belief, it appeared in interviews, was largely due to the greater success she had had in later years in avoiding serious tissue damage. Later evidence made it appear much more likely that this was due to more adult behaviour patterns, and to learning to use other cues as a warning of potentially damaging stimuli.

In other words she thought she was feeling at least some pain, merely because she did not get injured so often. Because she would, for instance, withdraw her hand from a flame and not leave it to get burnt, she assumed that the reason she withdrew it was that she was feeling pain. She would stop something sticking into her skin, and would think that the sensation she felt when it penetrated the skin was pain, because she wanted to be rid of it. The real reason she wanted to be rid of it would probably be that she thought that it was a sign of injury rather than that she disliked it for its own sake. She would realize that she was behaving in a similar way to other people in such situations, and because she had been taught that their behaviour meant that they were feeling pain, she could easily conclude that she too was feeling pain. She would be making an inference from her behaviour.

What, however, precisely would she be inferring? It seems as if she is concluding that she is feeling pain. This is what B. Aune[2] would maintain. He deals with what he considers to be the completely hypothetical case of someone who had never felt pain. He suggests that such a person could honestly claim to be in pain and be wrong. He says:

In relying, as he must, on behaviour that is accessible to all, his

---

[1] G. A. McMurray, *Archives of Neurology and Psychiatry*, 64 (1950), 654.
[2] *Philosophy in America*, ed. Max Black, p. 57.

statement faces the same risks as the statements that other people might make about him, or as the statements that he might make about the feelings of others.

Can anyone who is congenitally insensitive to pain be in as bad a position as this? Did the young woman have to infer from her behaviour whether she was feeling anything in the way in which she might infer from other people's behaviour that they were feeling something? Was she, in fact, in the same position as any observer of her behaviour? If she was, she clearly could make mistakes about what kind of sensation she was feeling. In extreme situations she would even make the mistake of thinking that she was feeling something when she was not, as this is a mistake which other people could make about her. A numb person might withdraw in apparent anguish from a flame, merely because he recognized it as a source of danger, and an observer might wrongly conclude that the man had felt pain.

Aune puts forward this view against that of Malcolm,[1] who maintains that the words 'I feel pain' cannot be used to state a conclusion. If someone who has never previously felt pain suddenly jumps and exclaims that he now does, Malcolm realizes that there is a temptation to ask how he recognized the new sensation as *pain*. He says:

Let us note that if the man gives an answer (e.g., 'I knew it must be pain because of the way I jumped') then he proves by that very fact that he has not mastered the correct use of the words 'I feel pain'. . . . In telling us how he did it he will convict himself of a misuse. Therefore the question 'How did he recognize his sensation?' requests the impossible.

Malcolm takes up this position because he cannot conceive what a mistake in identification of the sensation as pain would be. How would a situation where we recognize the sensation differ from one where we fail to, but think we do? What grounds could there be for prising apart a sincere avowal of a pain from the pain?

The young woman whose case we are considering apparently made an inference from her behaviour, namely that she was now feeling pain. Moreover, it was a mistaken one. Was she right in trying to use her behaviour as evidence for her

[1] *Journal of Philosophy*, 55 (1958), 977.

sensations? Aune would say she was. Malcolm, however, would hold that she was guilty of a gross misuse of the words 'I feel pain', which must always be spontaneous, according to him. Both seem to be asserting something true. The young woman did erroneously conclude something in connection with her behaviour. At the same time we do not require evidence to decide that we are feeling a sensation. We just feel it. We certainly do not make mistakes in feeling. There can be no difference between thinking that we feel something and actually feeling it.

This tells against Aune's view that the woman would be in the position of someone else observing her behaviour. This might be plausible if someone who had never felt pain had never felt anything. A numb person might make the basic conceptual error of thinking that being in pain was simply behaving in a certain way in appropriate situations without feeling anything. He might certainly then infer from his own behaviour that he had been in pain, if he caught himself withdrawing from a flame. This would be because he was basically mistaken over what 'pain' was. He would not mean the same by the word as other people. This would be shown by his failure to associate pain with feeling anything. It is significant that he could never make an inference from his behaviour to feeling pain. To him pain would not be something that could be felt.

The young woman was not numb, and would realize that 'pain' was the name of a sensation. Indeed Aune recognizes that the inference from behaviour is one to feeling pain. He does not think that someone who has never felt pain and who wrongly claims to feel it is committing any serious error about the concept. He wants to credit such a person 'with some understanding of what he says when he concludes that he must be feeling pain'. If then the young woman relied exclusively on her behaviour as a basis for her inference that she was feeling pain, it is clear that she was inferring two things. She was inferring that she was feeling something, and she was also inferring that what she felt was what other people called 'pain'. Both Aune and Malcolm run the two together and use arguments which are appropriate to one inference against the other.

The characteristic feature of an inference is not that it is a special kind of mental event which we can recognize as being an inference, instead of just being some kind of ordinary thought. It is rather a conclusion which we arrive at from something else. Could I infer that I am feeling a sensation or that what I am feeling is a sensation? The latter looks like an inference about the meaning of the word 'sensation'. The case we are interested in is one where we inferred that we were having a sensation (i.e. that we were feeling something), when we could not say spontaneously whether we were or not. We would conclude it from the way we were behaving. Our claim to feel something would in other words be based on evidence, and the evidence could be good or bad. We might be mistaken in our conclusion. This possibility is precisely what creates difficulties. What would it be to come to believe that one was feeling something and yet be wrong? How could the question of the presence or absence of a sensation be prised apart from my beliefs about it? It is impossible to talk of really feeling something when I think I am feeling nothing. If I believe that I am not feeling anything, then I am not feeling anything. It is self-contradictory to refer to a sensation and yet to say that I am not feeling it. We cannot talk of 'unnoticed sensations'. A sensation which I do not believe I am feeling is on a level with an unfelt sensation, and that is no sensation at all. Conversely if I think I am feeling something, then I must be feeling something. My beliefs about my sensations and my sensations themselves cannot be separated. There can be no difference between what seems to me to be so and what is so with regard to feelings. How could it ever be shown that my beliefs were incorrect?

We do talk of people changing their minds about what they felt, and this is usually a matter of their offering a description of the sensation which was different from the one they had given while they were feeling it. They may have revised their views about the application of a concept, and realized that their description was faulty because of a conceptual mistake. For example, someone might decide that he should not have called a sensation an 'itch', because he had had no inclination to scratch. If someone changed his mind not just about what to call the sensation, but about what exactly he had felt, there seems to be no reason why we should accept his second thoughts rather than his first. The fact that people's subsequent thoughts about a sensation differ from what they thought about it at the time does not offer an adequate basis for maintaining that a sensation can be different from what the person who has it thinks of it at the time.

In Chapter IV we quoted a puzzling case where, after hypnosis, a patient said he was not feeling any pain, at the same time as he wrote that he was. Both 'avowals' were apparently sincere. It seems that whether he was or was not feeling pain, at least some of his beliefs about it must be wrong. If he was in pain, what he said was wrong, and if he was not, what he wrote was wrong. It is, however, significant that, in the absence of any clear decision by the patient about whether he was feeling pain, we are unable to decide ourselves. We have already discussed possible ways of resolving the contradiction by disregarding one or other of the avowals, but this is very arbitrary. We are faced with criteria of equal validity both for the presence and for the absence of pain, and this means that we cannot make a decision. We can be in no better state than the patient. The case must remain completely perplexing. Although the patient could not have simultaneously felt pain and not felt it, we are in no position to say which is true. It is precisely because sensations cannot be prised apart from beliefs that we can make no decision. If it was possible to have erroneous, but sincere, beliefs about the presence of a sensation, it should be comparatively easy in this case to dismiss one set of beliefs as simply mistaken. The difficulty we have in doing this is a demonstration of the close relationship between beliefs and sensations.

The young woman who inferred from her growing ability to avoid injury that she was feeling pain was, according to Aune's account of that type of situation, inferring both that she was feeling something and that what she felt was 'pain'. We have seen that the first inference is an impossible one to make. We cannot believe that we are feeling something without feeling it, and yet the whole point of what Aune says is to show the possibility of a sincere claim to pain, which could be mistaken. Malcolm realizes that sensations cannot be inferred, and because of this denies that it is ever possible to infer that one is feeling pain. He does not examine the possibility of inferring that what is felt is to be called 'pain'. If it is possible to make a mistake over this, a sense can be given to an assertion that somebody wrongly inferred that he was in pain. This would not mean that the person inferred that he was feeling something when he was not feeling anything. It would not in fact be an inference to his feelings at all. It would be an inference to what to call his feelings. This would not be a case of a sensation being separated from the beliefs of the person who was having it. He would be under no doubt as to what kind of sensation it was, and he would certainly be under no doubt that he was feeling something.

The inference would be one about the extension of a concept. Indeed it might even be about what the concept was. In Chapter II[1] we noted that someone who knew what 'pain' meant might still be dubious as to whether to call electric shocks 'pains' or not. This would be a query about how far the concept of pain extends. The question would be whether we can allow for unpleasant sensations which are not pains. It might be argued that the fact he was not sure about the extension of the concept indicated that he did not have a complete grasp of it. Someone who had a clear idea of what pain was would know that not all unpleasant sensations were pains. Knowledge of a concept, however, is not an 'all or nothing' affair. Because a person is not sure about the extension of the concept in one instance, it does not follow that he is never sure. He may know that a whole range of sensations has something in common, and call them 'pains' as a result. If, however, he has always found them unpleasant, it would be natural for him to hesitate about what to call a similar sensation which was not unpleasant, or a dissimilar one which was. It is true that his hesitation is the result of the erroneous idea that a sensation's unpleasantness provides us with one of the reasons for calling it 'pain'. This is not a good enough reason for us to say sweepingly that his expression of doubt shows that he does not know what 'pain' means. He will use the word 'pain' appropriately in normal circumstances.

The young woman who was congenitally insensitive to pain would be in a worse position that this. She had never had occasion to say that she was in pain herself, although she would be able to recognize whether others were in pain as well as anybody else. Any decision she would have to make would not just be whether a certain type of sensation should be grouped with 'pains', but what a 'pain' was. What sensation did other people call 'pain'? Someone who hesitates about whether to

[1] p. 22.

call an electric shock 'pain' may be tempted to do so because of its unpleasantness. The fact that people do not very readily do so is because they recognize that the sensation feels noticeably different from the others which they call 'pain'. They know that the quality of the sensation is a relevant factor. The realization that this is so is essential for an adequate grasp of the concept. Anyone who had never felt pain would not necessarily have understood this much. Because they have not been able to learn the concept in a normal way, they will have to learn its nature from the situations in which people refer to 'pain'. It will not be surprising if they make mistakes about what kind of sensation other people call 'pain'. An obvious trap for them is to assume that it merely means 'an unpleasant sensation'. They can be warned of this mistake and of others, but the possibility of error is there. We can envisage someone who had never felt pain finding a sensation unpleasant and concluding that he felt 'pain'. He would be inferring that this is the kind of sensation which others call 'pain'. He might find nausea unpleasant and for that reason call it 'painful'. He would be concluding that he was in pain. That he was feeling something would not be the result of an inference. What he called it very definitely was.

Despite what Malcolm says, it is possible to infer that one is feeling pain and be wrong. It is an inference about the basis on which we call sensations 'pain'. This is not an unusual type of inference to make. We often have to make a decision, as a result of evidence which may be good or bad, as to what is the correct word to use on a certain occasion. Clearly the possibility of mistake is always with us in such circumstances. Anyone who has to talk in a foreign language is particularly vulnerable. A foreigner learning English might, for instance, notice that people often greeted each other by saying 'Hello'. He might, however, conclude that it was just a friendly form of address which could be used when parting from someone as well as when meeting them. He would soon get caught out when he said 'hello', when he should have said 'goodbye'. He would be wrong, and could be corrected.

4. *An Analogy with Colour-Blindness*

Someone who was colour-blind would be in a somewhat similar

position to anyone who could not feel pain. Just as the latter would have to conclude from evidence what sensations he should call 'pain' (assuming that he thought that he was starting to feel pain), so the former would conclude what colour-words he should apply to what objects. The most common form of colour-blindness is an inability to distinguish red from green. This would show itself in a failure to sort out red objects from green ones, if they were otherwise identical. Clearly, however, it would be possible for such a person to infer from an object's shape or purpose what colour it was, when he was faced with an array of different objects. He would not be able to infer how it looked to him. He could infer whether 'red' or 'green' was the right word to use. If, for example, he had been told that pillar-boxes were red, he would be able to say that a particular pillar-box was red, when he was confronted with it. Its colour might look no different to him from that of grass, but this would not prevent him from saying that the colour of pillar-boxes was red and that of grass green. He would be using the nature of the object as his guide as to what to call its colour, just as the woman who had felt no pain used her reaction to tell her whether she should call her sensation 'pain' or not. Both cases give rise to the same possibility of error. The man who was partially colour-blind would be caught out in Southern Ireland where pillar-boxes are identical with those in England but for the fact that they are green. The woman was misled by her assumption that any sensation which made her take action to avoid its cause (such as withdrawing her hand from the fire) must for that reason be called 'pain'.

The parallel must not be pressed too far. The colour-blind person is not making a conceptual mistake about the application of the word 'red'. He realizes, from his ability to use other colour words normally (apart from 'green'), that the shape or function of a thing does not provide adequate grounds for calling anything 'red', but he has to rely on them because of his disability. The person who has never felt pain, but now wants to say for one reason or another that he is feeling it, is in a different position. He lays himself open to making a basic error about how we apply the word 'pain' to sensations. If he fails to realize the importance of the quality of the sensation, he might easily call a sensation a 'pain', when it might transpire that it was merely a sensation he disliked or a sensation which made him avoid physical damage. In such a situation we could say that he was wrong in saying his sensation was a 'pain'. No one can refer to a sensation as a 'pain' without implying that it has something in common (other than the reaction) with other sensations which we also call 'pains'. If someone denies that they are implying this when they talk of 'pain', they thereby show that they have not a proper grasp of the concept.

We have in earlier chapters stressed the necessity for some assurance that a person who uses the word 'pain' in strange situations fully understands its meaning. There must be no possibility that he be in the same position as the young woman who could sincerely say that a sensation was 'pain' and yet be wrong, because of a faulty conception of what 'pain' is. If the concept had not been learned properly, there is the possibility of mistake. Once someone has learnt the concept of pain, no sense can be given to the question whether the sensation which they call 'pain' is really 'pain' or not. If they say it is the same as other sensations which they have called 'pain', then it is. As Wittgenstein indicates, we cannot get between their sensation and their description of it. This points to the difference between the person who is colour-blind and the person who feels no pain. It would be possible for the former to have a completely adequate concept of red. He would know it was a colour which he was unable to see properly, but he would be able to grasp the fact that red and green were different colours, just as, say, blue and yellow were different. He need not be convicted of any conceptual mistake, but he could still be wrong in calling an object 'red'. The man who has been congenitally insensitive to pain only has to demonstrate that he has learnt the concept for a statement by him that he is feeling 'pain' to be accepted.

Conventional 'pain-behaviour', such as writhing or moaning, is a sign of the presence of distress and not of pain. It provides an indispensable condition for the learning of the concept of pain, but it is dangerous to rely on such behaviour as providing rigid criteria for the presence of pain. We in fact have substituted a piece of verbal behaviour as the criterion of pain. The fact that it is incorrigible is a consequence of the recognition that no sense can be given to the possibility of wrongly identifying a sensation. We have made a full grasp of the concept, including a knowledge of the importance of the quality of pain, a pre-condition, since without it mistaken inferences can easily be made. The case of the young woman who was congenitally insensitive to pain and made such a mistake is an example of this.

BIBLIOGRAPHY

PART I—PHILOSOPHY

ANSCOMBE, G. E. M. 'The Intentionality of Sensation. A Grammatical Feature', *Analytical Philosophy* (second series), ed. R. J. Butler, Oxford, 1965.

ARMSTRONG, D. M. *Bodily Sensations*, London, 1962.

AUNE, B. 'On the Complexity of Avowals', *Philosophy in America*, ed. M. Black, London 1965.

BAIER, K. *The Moral Point of View*, Cornell, 1958.
'Pains', *Australasian Journal of Philosophy*, vol. 40, 1962.

BEDFORD, E. 'Emotions', *Proceedings of the Aristotelian Society*, vol. lvii, 1956–7.

BRADLEY, F. H. 'On Pleasure, Pain, Desire and Volition', *Mind*, vol. xiii, 1888.

BRENTANO, F. 'The Distinction between Mental and Physical Phenomena', *Realism and the Background of Phenomenology*, ed. R. M. Chisholm, Glencoe, Illinois, 1960.

BROAD, C. D. *Five Types of Ethical Theory*, London, 1930.
Examination of McTaggart's Philosophy, Cambridge, 1933.

BROWN, S. C. 'Intentionality Without Grammar', *Proceedings of the Aristotelian Society*, vol. lxv, 1964–5.

CHISHOLM, R. M. *Perceiving*, Cornell, 1957.

FEIBLEMAN, J. S. 'A Philosophical Analysis of Pleasure', *The Role of Pleasure in Behavior*, ed. R. G. Heath, New York, 1964.

GALLIE, W. B. 'Pleasure', *The Aristotelian Society, Supplementary Volume*, xxviii, 1954.

HAMPSHIRE, S. *Freedom of the Individual*, London, 1965.

HARE, R. M. 'Pain and Evil', *The Aristotelian Society, Supplementary Volume*, xxxviii, 1964.

HOSPERS, J. *Human Conduct*, London, 1963.

KENNY, A. *Action, Emotion and Will*, London, 1963.

MALCOLM, N. 'Knowledge of Other Minds,' *Journal of Philosophy*, vol. 55, 1958.

MANSER, A. R. 'Pleasure', *Proceedings of the Aristotelian Society*, vol. lxi, 1960–1.

MARSHALL, H. R. *Pain, Pleasure and Aesthetics*, London, 1894.

MOORE, G. E. *Commonplace Book*, London, 1963.

O'SHAUGHNESSY, R. J. 'Enjoying and Suffering', *Analysis*, vol. 26, 1966.

PITCHER, G. 'Emotion', *Mind*, vol. lxxiv, 1965.

RYLE, G. *The Concept of Mind*, London, 1949.

Dilemmas, Cambridge, 1954.

'Pleasure', *The Aristotelian Society, Supplementary Volume*, xxviii, 1954.

TAYLOR, C. C. W. 'Pleasure', *Analysis*, vol. 23, (Supplement), 1963.

VESEY, G. N. A. *The Embodied Mind*, London, 1965.

VON WRIGHT, G. *The Varieties of Goodness*, London, 1963.

WHITE, A. R. *Attention*, Oxford, 1965.

WITTGENSTEIN, L. *The Blue and Brown Books*, Oxford, 1958.

Philosophical Investigations (transl. G. E. M. Anscombe), 2nd ed., Oxford, 1958.

Zettel (transl. G. E. M. Anscombe), Oxford, 1967.

ZINK, S. *The Concepts of Ethics*, London, 1962.

PART II—MISCELLANEOUS

ARNOLD, M. B. *Emotion and Personality*, London 1961.

BARBER, T. X. 'Towards a Theory of Pain', *Psychological Bulletin*, vol. 56, 1959.

BAXTER, D. W. and OBSZEWSKI, J. 'Congenital Universal Insensitivity to Pain', *Brain*, vol. 83, 1960.

BEECHER, H. K. 'Pain in Men Wounded in Battle', *Annals of Surgery*, vol. 123, 1946.

Measurement of Subjective Responses, New York, 1959.

BISHOP, G. H. 'Neural Mechanisms of Cutaneous Sense', *Physiological Reviews*, vol. 26, 1946.

BONNER, F., COBB, S., SWEET, W. H. and WHITE, J. C. 'Frontal Lobe Surgery in the Treatment of Pain', *Psychosomatic Medicine*, vol. 14, 1952.

CHAPMAN, L. F., DINGMAN, H. F., and GINZBERG, S. P. 'Pain Thresholds and Analgesic Agents', *Brain*, vol. 88, 1965.

CRITCHLEY, M. 'Congenital Indifference to Pain', *Annals of Internal Medicine*, vol. 45, 1956.

EDWARDS, W. 'Recent Research on Pain Perception', *Psychological Bulletin*, vol. 47, 1950.

ELITHORN, A., GLITHERO, E., and SLATER, E. 'Leucotomy for Pain', *Journal of Neurology, Neurosurgery and Psychiatry*, vol. 21, N.S., 1958.

FALCONER, M. A. 'Relief of Intractable Pain of Organic Origin by Frontal Lobotomy', *Research Publications: Association for Research in Nervous and Mental Disease*, vol. xxvii, 1948.

FERENCZI, S. *Further Contributions to the Theory and Technique of Psychoanalysis*, transl., London, 1926.

FREEMAN, W. and WATTS, W. *Psychosurgery*, Springfield, 1950 (2nd ed.).

FREUD, S. 'The Economic Problem of Masochism', Standard Ed. 19, London, 1961.

GOMBRICH, E. H. *Art and Illusion*, London, 1960.

GOODY, W. 'On the Nature of Pain', *Brain*, vol. 80, 1957.

GÜTTMAN, E., and MAYER-CROSS, W. 'The Psychology of Pain', *Lancet*, February 1943.

HALL, K. R. L., and STRIDE, E. 'The Varying Response to Pain in Psychiatric Disorders', *British Journal of Medical Psychology*, vol. 27, 1954.

HARDY, J. D., WOLFF, H. G. and GOODELL, H. *Pain Sensations and Reactions*, Baltimore, 1952.

HEAD, H. *Studies in Neurology*, London, 1920.

HEMPHILL, R. E. and STENGEL, E. 'A Study on Pure Word-Deafness', *Journal of Neurology and Psychiatry*, vol. 3, N.S., 1940.

JEWSBURY, E. C. 'Insensitivity to Pain', *Brain*, vol. 74, 1951.

KAPLAN, E. A. 'Hypnosis and Pain', *Archives of General Psychiatry*, vol. 2, 1960.

KEATS, S. and BEECHER, H. K. 'Pain Relief with Hypnotic Doses of Barbiturates', *Journal of Pharmacology and Experimental Therapeutics*, vol. 100, 1950.

KEELE, C. A. and SMITH R. (ed.) *The Assessment of Pain in Man and Animals* (UFAW Symposium), London, 1962.

KEISER, S. 'The Fear of Sexual Passivity in the Masochist', *International Journal of Psycho-analysis*, vol. 30, 1949.

KOSKOFF, Y. D., DENNIS, W., LAZOVIK, D. and WHEELER, E. T. 'The Psychological Effects of Frontal Lobotomy, Performed for the Alleviation of Pain', *Res. Publ. Ass. nerv. ment. Dis.* vol. xxvii, 1948.

KUNKLE, E. C. and CHAPMAN, W. P. 'Insensitivity to Pain in Man', *Res. Publ. Ass. nerv. ment. Dis.* vol. xxiii, 1942.

LEWINSKY, H. 'On some Aspects of Masochism', *International Journal of Psychoanalysis*, vol 25, 1944.

McMURRAY, G. A. 'Experimental Study of a Case of Insensitivity to Pain', *Archives of Neurology and Psychiatry*, vol. 64, 1950.

NEMIAH, J. C. 'The Effect of Leucotomy on Pain', *Psychosomatic Medicine*, vol. 24, 1962.

OLDS, J. 'Self-Stimulation Experiments and Differentiated Reward Systems', *Motivation* (Penguin Modern Psychology), London 1966.

REIK, T. *Masochism in Modern Man*, transl. New York, 1957.

ROBINSON, M. F. and FREEMAN, W. *Psychosurgery and the Self*, New York, 1954.

RUBINS, J. L. and FRIEDMAN, E. D. 'Asymbolia for Pain', *Archives of Neurology and Psychiatry*, vol. 60, 1948.

SAUERBRUCH, F. and WENKE, H. *Pain, Its Meaning and Significance*, transl. E. Fitzgerald, London, 1963.

SCHNEIDER, S. F. 'A Psychological Basis for Indifference to Pain', *Psychosomatic Medicine*, vol. 24, 1962.

STEIN, M. H. 'The Problem of Masochism in the Theory and Technique of Psychoanalysis', *Journal of American Psychoanalytic Association*, vol. 4, 1956.

STERNBACH, R. A. 'Congenital Insensitivity to Pain', *Psychological Bulletin*, vol. 60, 1963.

STRONG, C. A. 'The Psychology of Pain', *Psychological Review*, vol. 2, 1895.

WATTS, W. and FREEMAN, W. 'Frontal Lobotomy in the Treatment of Unbearable Pain', *Res. Publ. Ass. nerv. ment. Dis.*, vol. 23, 1942.

WOLFF, H. G. and HARDY, J. D. 'The Nature of Pain', *Physiological Reviews*, vol. 27, 1947.

WOLFF, H. G., HARDY, J. D., and GOODELL, H. 'Studies on Pain', *Journal of Clinical Investigation*, vol 19, 1940.

WOLFF, H. G. and WOLF, S. *Pain*, 2nd Edn., Springfield, 1958.

INDEX

Ache, 39
Agony, 140 f.
Anger, 5 ff., 14 f.
Anscombe, G. E. M., 9 ff.
Anxiety, 5 f., 18, 74, 78, 97 f., 129 ff.,
   150
Aristotle, 121
Armstrong, D., 34 f., 39, 43 ff., 59,
   61, 125
Arnold, M. D., 4
Aspect Theory, 1, 4, 20, 34, 120, 124
Asymbolia for Pain, 69 ff., 126 f., 165
Attitude, 51 f.
Aune, B., 170 ff.

Baier, K., 64, 125
Beecher, H. K., 7, 55, 74 ff., 145
Bentham, J., 102
Bishop, G. H., 143 ff.
Bonner, F., 135, 137
Bradley, F. H., 1 f.
Brentano, F., 10 f., 36
Broad, C. D., 23 ff., 119 f., 122 f.

Chapman, L. F., 146 ff.
Chisholm, R. M., 9 ff.
Cobb, S., 135, 137
Colour, 27 f., 84 f.
Colour-blindness, 175 ff.
Concept
   the boundaries of a, 21
   the extension of a, 30 f.

Dennis, W., 127
Depression, 6
Dingman, H. F., 146 ff.
Discomfort, 2, 38 ff., 96, 147 f., 161 f.
Dislike, 52 ff., 116, 134 ff.
   and disapproval, 52
   and distress, 48, 56, 100 f., 115
Displeasure, 1 f., 20, 106
Distress, *passim*, especially 55 ff.
Duck-rabbit, 81 ff.

Eidelberg, L., 160 f.
Electric Shock, 22, 30, 54, 175

Elithorn, A., 133 f., 138
Emotion
   and agitation, 42, 49
   cause and object distinguished, 11,
      17 f., 159 f.
   duration of, 42 ff.
   and 'objects', 5 ff.
   and reasons, 50
   and viewing objects as good or bad,
      57
Enjoyment, 12, 119, 124, 151 ff., 157 f.

Falconer, M. A., 133, 135
Family Resemblance, 28 f.
Fear, 5 f., 51, 98 f., 115, 122
Feibleman, J. S., 120 f.
Ferenczi, S., 158
Forbes, A., 55, 145
Freeman, W., 126, 128, 130 f., 137 f.
Freud, S., 151 ff.
Friedman, E. D., 72 f.

Gallie, W. B., 107 f.
Ginzberg, S. P., 146 ff.
Glithero, E., 133 f., 138
Gombrich, E. H., 84
Hall, K. R. L., 68 f.
Hampshire, S., 51 f.
Hardy, J. D., 129
Head, H., 2, 22, 34
Headache, 28, 96 f., 123
Heath, R. G., 120
Hemphill, R. E., 70 f., 74
Hospers, J., 106 f., 159
'Hurt', 54 f.
Hypnosis, 66 f., 174
Identity
   of emotions, 98 ff.
   of pains, 87 ff.
   of sensations, 80 f., 87 ff., 91 ff.
Intensity
   and attention, 46 f.
   and dislike, 44, 139 ff.
   of emotions, 115
   and the evil of pain, 59
   of pain, 28, 150